Dr. Susan Lark's

Premenstrual Syndrome Self-Help Book

A WOMAN'S GUIDE TO FEELING GOOD ALL MONTH

Susan M. Lark, M.D.

The first completely practical, all-natural master plan for relieving over 150 symptoms of PMS

FORMAN PUBLISHING, INC. • LOS ANGELES

Design: Naomi Schiff
Illustration: Naomi Schiff and Kathie Klarreich
Photographs: Stephen Marley
Typesetting: Computer Typesetting Services
Printing: Dharma Press

Forman Publishing, Inc.
11661 San Vicente Blvd.
Los Angeles, California 90049

ISBN 0-936614-03-X
Library of Congress Catalog Number 84-080190

Printed in the United States of America

91 90 89 88 87 86 85 84   9 8 7 6 5 4 3 2

To Jim and Rebecca, with all my love

Contents

Acknowledgements

I am grateful to Jim, my husband, for his love and support; and to Gina Hakansson for her help and friendship when I was juggling a new baby, my medical practice, and authorship of this book.

Rose Bank, my consultant for the chapter on yoga, and Marcia Nelson, my consultant for the chapter on acupressure, helped greatly to make the book what it is. Adolph Smith, Ph.D., and David Lark, M.D., gave good advice, suggestions and support. Thanks are also due to: Luke Gatto for his inspiration and useful information on nutrition; B. K. Moran for editing the manuscript; Naomi Schiff for her art direction and production management; Nancy Friedman for copy editing and proofreading; and Judy Brand and Roxanne Kelly for their diligent and careful typing of the manuscript.

Finally, I want to thank my darling daughter Rebecca— my creativity sprang from her birth and the love I feel for her—and my patients, with appreciation and gratitude for all they have taught me.

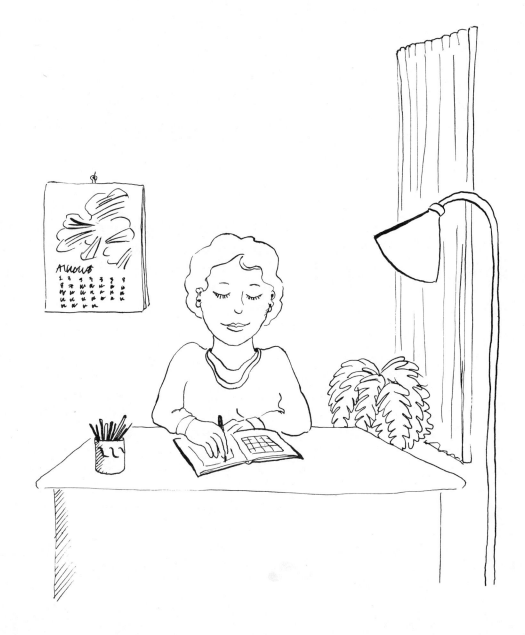

Introduction:
A Self-Help Approach
to Premenstrual Syndrome

Ten years ago, the serious symptoms suffered by millions of American women because of premenstrual syndrome were assumed by most of the medical profession and the rest of society to be part of a woman's nature and, thus, something she had to live with. What treatment medicine did have to offer was largely symptomatic and often ineffective.

Most doctors remained unaware of the accumulating body of medical research that described a variety of probable underlying metabolic causes of PMS. This research suggested that the metabolic imbalances could be relieved by changes in living habits: in nutrition, in patterns of work and exercise, and in ways of dealing with stress. Nine years ago, I began applying these ideas in my practice. Over the years I found that if I worked closely with my patients, together we could get better results than had ever seemed possible. Women who had missed work a week out of every month, who had been on the brink of hospitalization for emotional problems, whose family lives had been torn apart, were suddenly completely healthy and full of energy and good spirit. Seeing people's lives and health improve so radically through their own efforts is a wonderful experience, and I was eager to share it.

In the last few years great strides have been made in bringing information about PMS to public attention. Stories about PMS appear almost weekly on television, on the radio, and in newspapers and magazines. These stories have brought American women up to date on the symptoms of PMS, the wonderful new drugs for patients with more severe symptoms, and some general guidelines about nutrition and healthful habits of life. But they have been very sketchy in their treatment of the changes women need to make in order to prevent and relieve their symptoms. Even the current crop of books that purport to give self-help guidance are long on case histories and medical information and very short on the specific information women need to adapt their living habits through a PMS regimen.

My experience has been that once a woman realizes that her PMS symptoms can originate in bad habits of diet, exercise and management of stress, she is willing to do almost anything to change. But she needs specifics: guidelines, meal plans, recipes, stress reduction techniques, and the particular exercises from yoga, acupressure massage, and chiropractic that give direct relief of symptoms.

In working with my patients, I have gathered all this material. This book has been written so that I may share it with many more women than I could ever see in my practice. I hope that you will find it as helpful and enjoy using it as much as my patients and I have.

Learning to Cure Myself

I first found out about PMS during my late teens when I began to suffer from symptoms. My menstrual periods, which had always been irregular, began to be preceded by bloating and weight gain of five to eight pounds. My hair became oilier and little red pimples began to appear on my nose and chin.

During those years there was nothing for me to do except take aspirin. When I asked my mother for help she could only offer sympathy. She told me that I'd probably grow out of it as I got older. Instead, it got worse. My PMS continued all through my medical training at Northwestern University in Chicago. One week out of the month I was in too much pain to do my work properly. I still remember the many afternoons when I had to leave the medical or pediatric ward. I went to the medical student on-call room and lay there in agony with severe nausea and cramps. My body swelled up so badly that I couldn't bear to bump against anything. The cysts in my breasts became large and tender. I was the only woman student on many of my rotations and my symptoms made me feel inferior to and different from the male students. My moods fluctuated terribly. Part of the month I would feel calm and relaxed—like everyone else. But before my period I became quarrelsome and hard to deal with. I became much more sensitive to imagined or real slights and put-downs. I craved sugar and went on junk-food binges. Often I'd steal away and cry, not knowing how I was ever going to get through my training. I tried the accepted treatments—mild tranquilizers for my moods, antispasmodics for my cramps, and diuretics for my bloating. None of these medications worked particularly well.

Then, during my internship, everything changed. I was doing my specialty training in obstetrics and gynecology and was expected to keep up with the current medical research in my field. One day an article came across my desk. It described work being done by doctors in Europe who were using high doses of vitamins to treat breast cysts. Excited by this, I spent the rest of the year hunting in the medical library for other information about treating menstrual disorders through nutrition.

I began to test a very simple program on myself, using high doses of vitamin-B complex and vitamin E. Somewhat to my surprise, this helped my sugar craving, weight fluctuation, and bloating. Then I began to decrease the amount of sugar and caffeine in my diet. (As a busy student, I had depended on "quick energy" foods like sweet rolls and coffee. Medical students were expected to help take care of a large ward of sick patients on little sleep. We needed all the energy we could get, but mealtimes allowed for little more than grabbing a few bites in the cafeteria.) I began to pay more attention to my diet, eating more whole grains and fresh vegetables. I was amazed with the results: each month my premenstrual symptoms were less severe. However, my cyclical breast pain and mood swings persisted. A year later I learned from a journal article that Ovrette, a synthetic progesterone-like hormone, could be used to counteract symptoms—including water retention—caused by an overabundance of estrogen. I tried it, and my breast pain and lumps disappeared. The major side effect was a greater tendency toward oily skin, oily hair, and pimples. I stayed on Ovrette for two years.

During my third year of self-treatment I learned to treat my mood swings and irritability with biofeedback and other stress reduction techniques. Today I am totally free of premenstrual symptoms.

Learning to Work Together with My Patients

I was my first successful PMS patient. In the last nine years, I've treated hundreds of women with the problem, first in my family practice and then in the clinical program I started in Mountain View especially for women with PMS. In this program the physicians worked together with psychologists, a chiropractor, and a nutritionist in an integrative approach to health care. I also learned acupressure massage techniques and yoga positions in order to use them with my patients.

Together with these practitioners, we found that a number of methods can work to correct the symptoms of PMS. Western medicine provides symptomatic relief through medication and hormones. It also offers longer-term correction through nutrition and stress reduction. Acupressure massage, body work, chiropractic, and herbology also offer help that can be so immediate it seems almost miraculous to the patient. My patients today do not have to wait years, as I did, to see their symptoms disappear. Most of them feel outstandingly better in one to three months.

How a Self-Help Approach Can Work for You

PMS doesn't hit a victim at random like a thunderbolt. It is a metabolic imbalance that occurs slowly over the years because of our habits. Medication and therapeutic hormones can make you feel well very rapidly (as soon as thirty minutes after taking progesterone). But even women who have done beautifully on medical therapy find that their symptoms return when they stop medication if they haven't made substantial changes in their life habits.

This is why self-help can be so important. We are leaving the era when patients went passively to doctors looking for "magic pills." The patients gave up control of their problem to the doctor. This was not good for the doctor or the patient. Health care should be a team effort. People should be informed as to the choices available and the physician should function as an educator as well as provide loving care and support.

Self-help means that you take responsibility for your own health. Taking responsibility will make you stronger and give you confidence. It will help you to build a record of success (wellness) instead of failure and illness. Self-help tools like nutrition and stress reduction have less potential for harmful side effects than drugs do. They are safer and gentler methods.

As I mentioned, I work with many self-help methods. A treatment plan that utilizes only one method and purports to be *the* treatment for PMS will probably work for only a small percentage of women. I have found that my results are much better if I completely individualize each patient's treatment program. By overlapping treatments for various disciplines most women find a combination that works for them. There will be a combination that works for you too.

This program is set up so that you can individualize a treatment plan for yourself. All the methods you need are contained in this book. They include nutrition, stress reduction, exercise, acupressure massage, chiropractic exercises, and yoga. Read through the entire book first to familiarize yourself with the material. The PMS Workbook (Chapter Three) will help you evaluate your symptoms and the Complete Treatment Chart for PMS (Chapter Four) will tell you which treatments to use for your particular set of symptoms. Together they are quick and easy to use and will save you countless hours of work on your own.

What will work for you can be found simply and quickly. Try all of the therapies listed under your symptoms. You will probably find that some make you feel better than others. Establish a regimen that works for you and use it each month.

This program is easy to follow and practical. It can be used by itself or in conjunction with a medical program. And best of all, it works. The feeling of wellness that can be yours with a self-help program will radiate out and touch your whole life. You will have more time and energy to enjoy your work, family, and other pleasures in life.

Part One:
The Problem

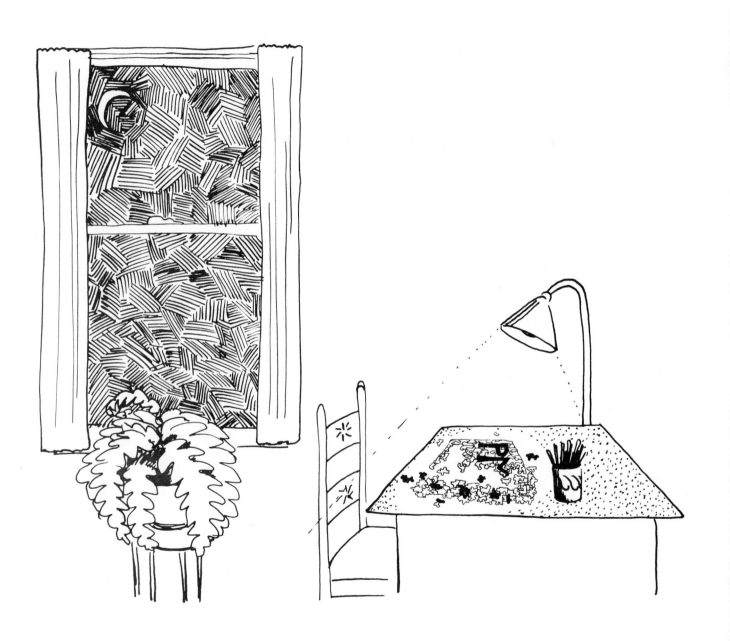

1

What Is Premenstrual Syndrome?

Premenstrual syndrome is one of the commonest problems affecting younger women. It is believed to affect between one third and one half of all American women between the ages of twenty and fifty—in other words, as many as ten to fourteen million women.

The symptoms usually begin ten to fourteen days prior to the onset of the menstrual period and become progressively worse until the onset of menstruation or, for some women, several days after the onset. This means that millions of women go through half of each month of their adult lives feeling sick. What this translates into in terms of lost productivity and quality of life is staggering.

The Symptoms

The symptoms of premenstrual syndrome (PMS) are numerous and affect almost every organ system of the body. More than 150 have been documented. Some of the most common ones are:

irritability	acne
anxiety	boils
mood swings	allergies
depression	hives
hostility	cystitis
migraine	urethritis
headache	less frequent urination
dizziness	asthma
fainting	breast tenderness and swelling
tremulousness	rhinitis
abdominal bloating	sore throat
weight gain	hoarseness
constipation	joint pain and swelling
sugar craving	backache
cramps	

It is common for many of these symptoms to co-exist in the same women. Patients often report as many as ten or twelve symptoms. PMS seems to touch every aspect of their lives—from their relationships with family and friends, to their work productivity, to their ability to take pleasure in their own bodies.

There is a pervasive sense of "things always falling apart" during the PMS period. Dr. Katharina Dalton, an English physician with extensive experience in treating women with premenstrual syndrome, noted that severely afflicted women are most vulnerable to extremes of behavior during this period. She documented an increased likelihood of accidents, alcohol abuse, suicide attempts, and crimes being committed by some women.

Although I rarely have patients who demonstrate such extreme aberrations, many do describe undergoing severe personality changes. They often describe Dr. Jekyll–and–Mr. Hyde personality splits. They say that they are "irritable," "witchy," and "mean"—that they yell at their children, pick fights with their spouses and snap at friends and co-workers. They often spend the rest of the month repairing the emotional damage done to their relationships during this time. Often their children are bewildered and hurt, not understanding how Mommy can suddenly turn so mean.

Until recently, these women would turn to their physicians for help and would be offered only a tranquilizer or a psychiatric referral. Women would invest time and money in counseling that often didn't help. This would only add to their sense of failure and confusion about their medical problem. Fortunately, the attitude of the medical profession is beginning to change. As the women's self-help movement grows and the problem continues to be publicized, more research is being undertaken to improve our understanding of the causes of this problem.

The Factors That Increase Your Risk

You are at increased risk of having PMS if:

- You are over thirty. (The most severe symptoms occur in women in their thirties and forties.)

- There is significant emotional stress in your life.

- You have the nutritional habits that contribute to PMS.

- You have suffered side effects from birth control pills. (Women who are unable to tolerate the pill seem to be more likely to get PMS.)

- You have difficulty maintaining a stable weight.

- You do not exercise.

- You are married.

- You have had a pregnancy complicated by toxemia.

- You have children. (The more children, the more severe the symptoms.)

2

The Causes and Types of PMS

THE NORMAL MENSTRUAL CYCLE

It is important that you understand how the normal menstrual cycle works. This knowledge will make it much easier for you to understand the changes your body chemistry undergoes with PMS.

The Purpose of Menstruation

Menstruation is the shedding of the lining of the uterus. With most women, this occurs each month. The lining of the uterus (the endometrium) increases in thickness throughout the monthly cycle due to an increase in the blood supply and micronutrients. This thickening occurs to prepare a home for the fertilized egg during its nine months of growth and development within the mother's uterus. If pregnancy does not occur, then this lining is not needed. The uterus cleanses itself of the cells with the monthly bleeding. It then prepares the endometrium all over again the following month.

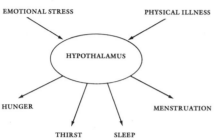

The Hormonal Feedback System

A cyclical pattern occurs because of the fluctuations in your hormonal levels. This is based on a feedback system in which the hormonal gland secretes a chemical (hormone), which enters the bloodstream and triggers a reaction in another gland far away. The hormone acts as a messenger, either giving another gland instructions to make its own hormone or triggering a chemical response in other parts of the body.

The menstrual cycle is triggered by hormones produced in the hypothalamus, a glandular center located in the brain above the pituitary. From this central location, it receives and sends nerve signals to many other parts of the brain. It regulates many functions, including hunger, thirst, sleep patterns, and all the endocrine functions, including menstruation. The hypothalamus is very sensitive to environmental stimuli such as emotional stress and physical illness. Such stress can modify the signals that the hypothalamus passes on to the pituitary and from there on to the rest of the endocrine system. This can cause irregularities in the menstrual cycle.

The hypothalamus communicates with the pituitary gland by releasing into the bloodstream messengers called FSH-RF (follicle-stimulating hormone-releasing factor) and LH-RF (luteinizing hormone-releasing factor). Their job is to tell the pituitary to make its own hormones.

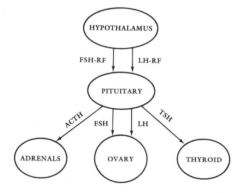

From its position at the base of the brain, just below the hypothalamus, the pituitary produces the hormones needed to stimulate all the other glands of the body. Thus it has a very important regulating function. It stimulates the menstrual cycle by producing FSH (follicle-stimulating hormone) and LH (luteinizing hormone) as well as adrenocorticotropic hormone (ACTH) and thyroid-stimulating hormone (TSH).

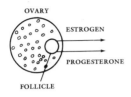

OVARY

ESTROGEN

PROGESTERONE

FOLLICLE

FSH and LH are released into the bloodstream with the ovaries as their destination. The ovaries are located in the woman's pelvic region and contain all the eggs that she will ever have. At birth each woman has between 100,000 and 400,000 eggs in an inactive form called follicles. They decrease progressively throughout her life until she reaches menopause, at which time most have been destroyed and the ovaries cease to function.

Each month, FSH and LH from the pituitary cause the follicles to ripen and one of them to grow into an egg. In doing so the follicle begins to produce the hormones estrogen and progesterone. Besides preparing the egg to be fertilized, these hormones also stimulate the lining of the uterus to prepare a proper home for the egg to grow. The estrogen and progesterone also control the obvious physical signs of femininity, such as breast development and growth of pubic hair. Sexual hormones in smaller amounts are also produced by the adrenal glands, which are located on top of the kidneys.

As estrogen and progesterone circulate through the bloodstream they pass through the liver. The liver functions as a garbage disposal service. When high levels of hormones are no longer needed, it breaks them down and renders them chemically inactive so that they can be excreted from the body. The kidney then excretes the chemically altered hormones into the urine and their passage through the body is complete.

The Monthly Cycle

On day 1, the first day of menstruation, estrogen and progesterone levels are extremely low. The hypothalamus reacts by releasing FSH-RF, which stimulates the pituitary to produce FSH. FSH stimulates the follicle cells of the ovary to

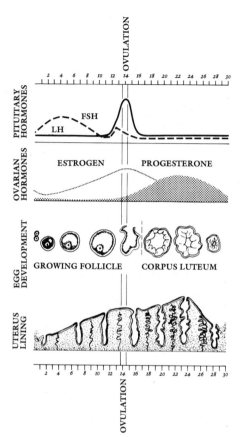

begin increasing in size and producing estrogen. The increased amounts of estrogen produced by these follicles stimulate the lining of the uterus to grow so that by midcycle it has increased three times in thickness and has a greatly increased blood supply.

One of the follicles, the Graafian follicle, surpasses the growth of the others and produces the egg for that month. At midcycle (day 14) and immediately prior to ovulation, estrogen levels reach their peak. This causes the pituitary to decrease the amount of FSH produced and increase the amount of LH. This triggers the release of the egg from the follicle and its extrusion from the ovary.

The egg is picked up by the Fallopian tube and stays there for twelve to thirty-six hours. It is during this time that the egg can be fertilized. Between midcycle and day 28, the LH causes the Graafian follicle left in the ovary to change into a corpus luteum, or yellow body. This yellow body produces high levels of estrogen and especially progesterone. Adequate levels of progesterone are essential for maintaining a pregnancy. Progesterone causes the increase in basal body temperature seen at ovulation. It also causes a coiling of the blood vessels of the endometrium so that the lining becomes more compact.

THE TYPES OF PMS

The most common symptoms of which PMS patients complain can be broken down into four subgroups according to the classification system developed by Dr. Guy Abraham, former clinical professor of obstetrics and gynecology at UCLA, who has published extensively on the subject of PMS.

Type A (for "anxiety"): anxiety, irritability, mood swings

Type C (for "carbohydrates" or "cravings"): sugar craving, fatigue, headaches

Type H (for "hyperhydration"): bloating, weight gain, breast tenderness

Type D (for "depression"): depression, confusion, memory loss

Added to these are two other common subgroups.

Acne: pimples, oily skin and hair

Dysmenorrhea: cramps, low back pain, nausea, and vomiting. Many doctors do not consider dysmenorrhea a part of PMS. But because it's such a common and debilitating symptom, I've included it and given therapies for it.

At the present time, the available medical research indicates that each symptom group is due to its own specific chemical imbalance. Thus, PMS may be looked upon as six different problem entities, often coexisting in the same woman. Let us look at each one of these subgroups separately.

Type A: Anxiety, Irritability and Mood Swings. Type A is the most common subtype. Abraham found that symptoms of anxiety, irritability, and mood swings occurred in 80 percent of the women he studied. In some women anxiety is followed by depression. The symptoms worsen in the days prior to the menstrual period and are relieved only with its onset.

The most likely cause of these symptoms is an imbalance in the body's estrogen and progesterone levels. Both estrogen

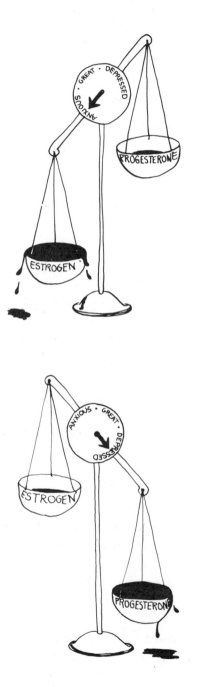

and progesterone increase during the second half of the menstrual cycle. Through their chemical action, they affect the function of almost every one of the body's organ systems. When properly balanced, estrogen and progesterone promote normal function of the uterus, vagina, and breast. PMS mood symptoms occur if the balance between these hormones is abnormal. This is because they have an opposing effect on the chemistry of the brain. If estrogens predominate, women tend to feel anxious. If progesterone predominates, women tend to feel depressed. (Other examples of the complementarity of estrogen and progesterone include the following: estrogen lowers blood sugar, progesterone elevates it; estrogen promotes synthesis of fats in the tissues, progesterone breaks them down.)

When estrogen and progesterone are appropriately balanced, women have normal moods and behavioral patterns. The balance between these hormones depends on two things: how much hormone is produced and how the hormone is disposed of. As I mentioned earlier, when the hormones have finished their metabolic tasks, they are brought to the liver and prepared for excretion by the kidney. Any breakdown in this system at any step will affect the hormonal balance. Both emotional stress and nutritional habits play significant roles in how efficiently this system will run. For example, foods that are too rich, such as excess fats and sugar, will overwork the liver, which must process them as well as the hormones. With vitamin B deficiency, which can be caused either by poor nutrition or by emotional stress, the liver does not have the raw material that it needs to carry out its metabolic tasks. In either case, the liver is unable to break down the hormones efficiently. This can increase the levels of estrogen or progesterone that continue to circulate in the blood without proper disposal.

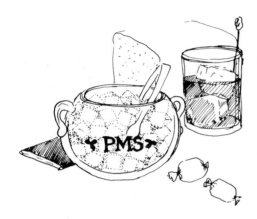

Type C: Sugar Craving, Fatigue, and Headaches. Sixty percent of women with PMS note an increased craving for refined carbohydrates, particularly sugar, chocolate, alcohol, white bread, pastries, white rice, and noodles. These women tend to eat much larger quantities of these foods before their periods than they normally would. This craving is much worse when women are under stress. A few hours after indulging in sweets, many complain of fatigue, headaches, shakiness, and dizziness.

Several mechanisms for the problem have been postulated. A woman's body is more responsive to insulin the week before her period starts. This tends to lower her blood sugar level because the insulin allows sugar to leave the bloodstream and enter the cells. With less circulating glucose, there is less sugar available for the brain, which uses up to twenty percent of the body's total energy supply. Glucose is the major energy form, or fuel, of the body. The brain signals that more fuel is needed, and the body translates that signal into an increased craving for sweets. This craving is worse if she is under stress, because her brain then needs more fuel. It is also worse if her nutritional habits are poor and she lacks sufficient vitamin B and magnesium in her diet. Without these nutrients, the body can't break down the sugar to use it for fuel.

In the premenstrual period many women crave chocolate and consume large quantities of it. Chocolate is fairly rich in magnesium. It is also rich in phenylethylamine, which has an antidepressant effect (remember, depression is very common with PMS). Chocolate craving may represent the body's need to find sources of nutrients that it is deficient in, but unfortunately, chocolate contains a number of ingredients that worsen PMS.

EXCESS ACTH

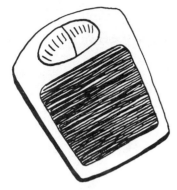

**FLUID AND
SODIUM RETENTION**

BLOATING

WEIGHT GAIN

BREAST TENDERNESS

EXCESS ANDROGENS

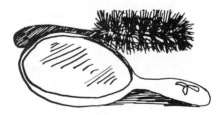

CHANGES PH OF SKIN

INCREASES OIL SECRETION

ACNE

Type H: Bloating, Weight Gain and Breast Tenderness.
Women with Type H complain of abdominal bloating, breast tenderness, and weight gain. Often the subjective sensation of bloating is worse than the actual weight gain, which is seldom more than three pounds. These women tend to retain excess fluid and salt. This is caused by an excess secretion of the pituitary hormone ACTH. ACTH is secreted by the pituitary and then is sent to the adrenal glands via the blood stream. The adrenals then secrete their own hormones which are sent to the kidneys. The kidney in response retains salt and water, so less urine is excreted. This means that you urinate less frequently. Forty percent of women with PMS experience these symptoms.

Type D: Depression, Confusion, Insomnia, and Memory Loss.
Type D is the least common form that Abraham identified. It is seen by itself in only 5 percent of women affected. In conjunction with Type A, it is seen in 20 percent.

Estrogen levels have been found to be low in women with Type D. Thus the depressant effects of high or normal progesterone are not counterbalanced by estrogen. Type D is potentially the most serious type of all because the women affected can be suicidal in severe cases. The depression also makes these women likely to become withdrawn, so that they are less likely to seek medical care.

Acne: Pimples and Oily Skin and Hair. Some women experience an increase in male hormones (androgens) from the adrenal gland in the time before their periods. This causes changes in the pH of the skin as well as an increase in the skin's oil secretion. Lesions may be found on the face, shoulders and back of susceptible women. Acne can go through three stages. Blackheads are the mildest lesions. They occur when skin pores are blocked by oil. Most of the oil in the pore is white, but the oil that is exposed to the air on the skin surface turns black. Whiteheads are the second stage of acne. With this stage, the oil has no pore opening to the outside. Drainage cannot occur. Cysts form underneath the skin and become infected. This environment is perfect for the overgrowth of the bacteria that cause the third stage, cystic acne. These appear as red blotches on the skin. The cysts are hard and deep and can be painful to touch. Cystic acne often causes the sufferer much mental anguish; it is difficult to treat and looks unattractive.

Dysmenorrhea: Cramps, Low Back Pain, Nausea and Vomiting. Cramps are often a young woman's introduction to discomfort surrounding the menstrual period. "Primary" (nonpathological) dysmenorrhea often begins during the teenage years. It is thought to be due to spasm of the uterine muscles. Pains can occur in the lower abdomen, lower back, or inner thighs. Dysmenorrhea was one of the commonest reasons, second only to colds, that young girls were excused from classroom attendance when I was a teenager. Research has found that primary dysmenorrhea is due to an imbalance in local chemicals produced by the uterus. These are called prostaglandins. There are nine subgroups of prostaglandins. In women without menstrual cramps the different prostaglandins are properly balanced. When there is an excess of prostaglandin F (which causes cramping and pain) over prostaglandin E, cramps are the result.

Secondary dysmenorrhea may occur in women over thirty. It may be due in part to mechanical problems such as fibroid tumors. Pelvic inflammatory infections and endometriosis can cause scar tissue in the pelvic region. This can cause painful stretching with the onset of menses. Congestion caused by retention of fluid and sodium may also worsen pelvic pain.

EXCESS PROSTAGLANDINS

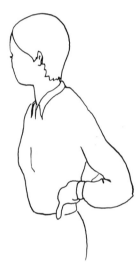

LOW BACK PAIN

CRAMPS

NAUSEA

VOMITING

Part Two:
Evaluating Your Symptoms

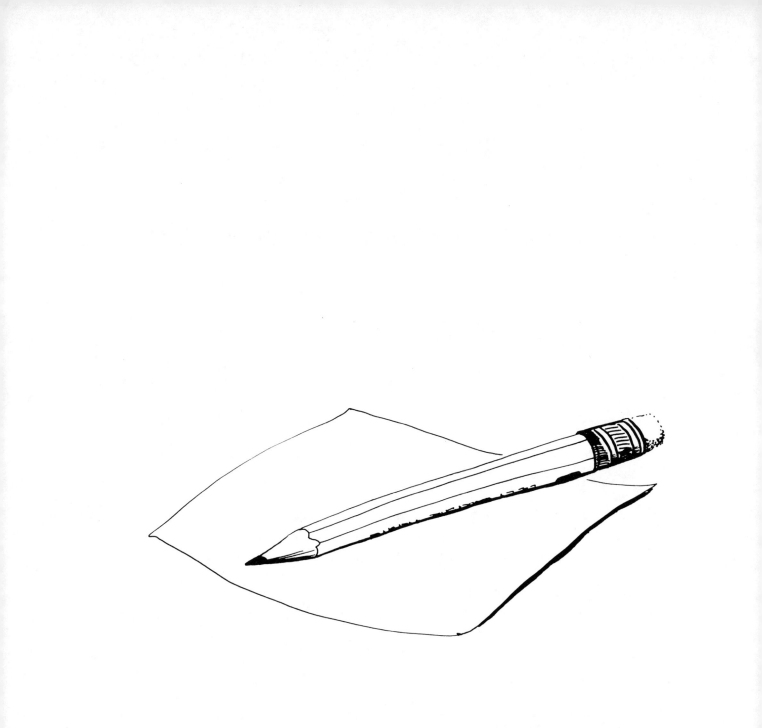

3

The PMS Workbook

EVALUATING YOUR SYMPTOMS

The evaluations on the next few pages will help you become more familiar with your own symptoms of PMS. If you take the time to fill them out, you'll find that they make it easy for you to identify your symptoms, recognize your weak areas, and put together your own treatment program from the chapters that follow.

First, fill out the monthly calendar of menstrual symptoms, starting with today. The calendar will allow you to classify your symptoms and see whether they cluster around a particular type or types. This will make it easier for you to pick the specific treatments for your symptoms. Then, as you follow the program, you can keep using the monthly calendars (a year's worth have been included) to check your progress.

After you've filled out the calendar for today, turn to the evaluations that follow the calendar section. They will help you assess specific areas of your life to see which of your habit patterns are contributing to your PMS.

When you've completed the evaluations, you will be ready to go on to Part Three and begin your treatment program.

Grade your symptoms as you experience them each month:

☐ None   ⊡ Mild   ◪ Moderate   ■ Severe

DAY OF CYCLE	1	2	3	4	5	6	7	8	9	10	11	12	13	14	15	16	17	18	19	20	21	22	23	24	25	26	27	28	29	30	31	32	33	34	35
TYPE A																																			
nervous tension																																			
mood swings																																			
irritability																																			
anxiety																																			
TYPE C																																			
headache																																			
craving for sweets																																			
increased appetite																																			
pounding heart																																			
fatigue																																			
tremulousness																																			
TYPE D																																			
depression																																			
forgetfulness																																			
crying																																			
sleeplessness																																			
TYPE H																																			
weight gain																																			
swelling of extremities																																			
breast tenderness																																			
abdominal bloating																																			
DYSMENORRHEA																																			
cramps (low abdominal)																																			
backache																																			
general aches and pains																																			
nausea and vomiting																																			
ACNE																																			
oily skin																																			
oily hair																																			
pimples																																			

Grade your symptoms as you experience them each month:

☐ *None*   ⊡ *Mild*   ◪ *Moderate*   ■ *Severe*

DAY OF CYCLE	1	2	3	4	5	6	7	8	9	10	11	12	13	14	15	16	17	18	19	20	21	22	23	24	25	26	27	28	29	30	31	32	33	34	35
TYPE A																																			
nervous tension																																			
mood swings																																			
irritability																																			
anxiety																																			
TYPE C																																			
headache																																			
craving for sweets																																			
increased appetite																																			
pounding heart																																			
fatigue																																			
tremulousness																																			
TYPE D																																			
depression																																			
forgetfulness																																			
crying																																			
sleeplessness																																			
TYPE H																																			
weight gain																																			
swelling of extremities																																			
breast tenderness																																			
abdominal bloating																																			
DYSMENORRHEA																																			
cramps (low abdominal)																																			
backache																																			
general aches and pains																																			
nausea and vomiting																																			
ACNE																																			
oily skin																																			
oily hair																																			
pimples																																			

MONTHLY CALENDAR OF MENSTRUAL SYMPTOMS

MONTH 3

Grade your symptoms as you experience them each month:

☐ None ⊡ Mild ◪ Moderate ■ Severe

DAY OF CYCLE	1	2	3	4	5	6	7	8	9	10	11	12	13	14	15	16	17	18	19	20	21	22	23	24	25	26	27	28	29	30	31	32	33	34	35
TYPE A																																			
nervous tension																																			
mood swings																																			
irritability																																			
anxiety																																			
TYPE C																																			
headache																																			
craving for sweets																																			
increased appetite																																			
pounding heart																																			
fatigue																																			
tremulousness																																			
TYPE D																																			
depression																																			
forgetfulness																																			
crying																																			
sleeplessness																																			
TYPE H																																			
weight gain																																			
swelling of extremities																																			
breast tenderness																																			
abdominal bloating																																			
DYSMENORRHEA																																			
cramps (low abdominal)																																			
backache																																			
general aches and pains																																			
nausea and vomiting																																			
ACNE																																			
oily skin																																			
oily hair																																			
pimples																																			

Grade your symptoms as you experience them each month:

☐ None   ⊡ Mild   ◸ Moderate   ■ Severe

DAY OF CYCLE	1	2	3	4	5	6	7	8	9	10	11	12	13	14	15	16	17	18	19	20	21	22	23	24	25	26	27	28	29	30	31	32	33	34	35
TYPE A																																			
nervous tension																																			
mood swings																																			
irritability																																			
anxiety																																			
TYPE C																																			
headache																																			
craving for sweets																																			
increased appetite																																			
pounding heart																																			
fatigue																																			
tremulousness																																			
TYPE D																																			
depression																																			
forgetfulness																																			
crying																																			
sleeplessness																																			
TYPE H																																			
weight gain																																			
swelling of extremities																																			
breast tenderness																																			
abdominal bloating																																			
DYSMENORRHEA																																			
cramps (low abdominal)																																			
backache																																			
general aches and pains																																			
nausea and vomiting																																			
ACNE																																			
oily skin																																			
oily hair																																			
pimples																																			

Grade your symptoms as you experience them each month:

☐ None   ⊡ Mild   ◨ Moderate   ■ Severe

DAY OF CYCLE	1 2 3 4 5 6 7 8 9 10 11 12 13 14 15 16 17 18 19 20 21 22 23 24 25 26 27 28 29 30 31 32 33 34 35
TYPE A	
nervous tension	
mood swings	
irritability	
anxiety	
TYPE C	
headache	
craving for sweets	
increased appetite	
pounding heart	
fatigue	
tremulousness	
TYPE D	
depression	
forgetfulness	
crying	
sleeplessness	
TYPE H	
weight gain	
swelling of extremities	
breast tenderness	
abdominal bloating	
DYSMENORRHEA	
cramps (low abdominal)	
backache	
general aches and pains	
nausea and vomiting	
ACNE	
oily skin	
oily hair	
pimples	

Grade your symptoms as you experience them each month:

☐ None   ⊡ Mild   ◪ Moderate   ■ Severe

DAY OF CYCLE	1	2	3	4	5	6	7	8	9	10	11	12	13	14	15	16	17	18	19	20	21	22	23	24	25	26	27	28	29	30	31	32	33	34	35
TYPE A																																			
nervous tension																																			
mood swings																																			
irritability																																			
anxiety																																			
TYPE C																																			
headache																																			
craving for sweets																																			
increased appetite																																			
pounding heart																																			
fatigue																																			
tremulousness																																			
TYPE D																																			
depression																																			
forgetfulness																																			
crying																																			
sleeplessness																																			
TYPE H																																			
weight gain																																			
swelling of extremities																																			
breast tenderness																																			
abdominal bloating																																			
DYSMENORRHEA																																			
cramps (low abdominal)																																			
backache																																			
general aches and pains																																			
nausea and vomiting																																			
ACNE																																			
oily skin																																			
oily hair																																			
pimples																																			

Grade your symptoms as you experience them each month:

☐ None　　● Mild　　◪ Moderate　　■ Severe

DAY OF CYCLE　　1　2　3　4　5　6　7　8　9　10　11　12　13　14　15　16　17　18　19　20　21　22　23　24　25　26　27　28　29　30　31　32　33　34　35

TYPE A

nervous tension

mood swings

irritability

anxiety

TYPE C

headache

craving for sweets

increased appetite

pounding heart

fatigue

tremulousness

TYPE D

depression

forgetfulness

crying

sleeplessness

TYPE H

weight gain

swelling of extremities

breast tenderness

abdominal bloating

DYSMENORRHEA

cramps (low abdominal)

backache

general aches and pains

nausea and vomiting

ACNE

oily skin

oily hair

pimples

MONTHLY CALENDAR OF MENSTRUAL SYMPTOMS

Grade your symptoms as you experience them each month:

☐ *None*   ▪ *Mild*   ◪ *Moderate*   ■ *Severe*

DAY OF CYCLE	1 2 3 4 5 6 7 8 9 10 11 12 13 14 15 16 17 18 19 20 21 22 23 24 25 26 27 28 29 30 31 32 33 34 35
TYPE A	
nervous tension	
mood swings	
irritability	
anxiety	
TYPE C	
headache	
craving for sweets	
increased appetite	
pounding heart	
fatigue	
tremulousness	
TYPE D	
depression	
forgetfulness	
crying	
sleeplessness	
TYPE H	
weight gain	
swelling of extremities	
breast tenderness	
abdominal bloating	
DYSMENORRHEA	
cramps (low abdominal)	
backache	
general aches and pains	
nausea and vomiting	
ACNE	
oily skin	
oily hair	
pimples	

Grade your symptoms as you experience them each month:

☐ None   ⊡ Mild   ◩ Moderate   ■ Severe

DAY OF CYCLE	1	2	3	4	5	6	7	8	9	10	11	12	13	14	15	16	17	18	19	20	21	22	23	24	25	26	27	28	29	30	31	32	33	34	35
TYPE A																																			
nervous tension																																			
mood swings																																			
irritability																																			
anxiety																																			
TYPE C																																			
headache																																			
craving for sweets																																			
increased appetite																																			
pounding heart																																			
fatigue																																			
tremulousness																																			
TYPE D																																			
depression																																			
forgetfulness																																			
crying																																			
sleeplessness																																			
TYPE H																																			
weight gain																																			
swelling of extremities																																			
breast tenderness																																			
abdominal bloating																																			
DYSMENORRHEA																																			
cramps (low abdominal)																																			
backache																																			
general aches and pains																																			
nausea and vomiting																																			
ACNE																																			
oily skin																																			
oily hair																																			
pimples																																			

Grade your symptoms as you experience them each month:

☐ *None*   ⊡ *Mild*   ◪ *Moderate*   ◼ *Severe*

DAY OF CYCLE	1	2	3	4	5	6	7	8	9	10	11	12	13	14	15	16	17	18	19	20	21	22	23	24	25	26	27	28	29	30	31	32	33	34	35
TYPE A																																			
nervous tension																																			
mood swings																																			
irritability																																			
anxiety																																			
TYPE C																																			
headache																																			
craving for sweets																																			
increased appetite																																			
pounding heart																																			
fatigue																																			
tremulousness																																			
TYPE D																																			
depression																																			
forgetfulness																																			
crying																																			
sleeplessness																																			
TYPE H																																			
weight gain																																			
swelling of extremities																																			
breast tenderness																																			
abdominal bloating																																			
DYSMENORRHEA																																			
cramps (low abdominal)																																			
backache																																			
general aches and pains																																			
nausea and vomiting																																			
ACNE																																			
oily skin																																			
oily hair																																			
pimples																																			

Grade your symptoms as you experience them each month:

☐ **None**   ⊡ **Mild**   ◨ **Moderate**   ■ **Severe**

DAY OF CYCLE	1	2	3	4	5	6	7	8	9	10	11	12	13	14	15	16	17	18	19	20	21	22	23	24	25	26	27	28	29	30	31	32	33	34	35
TYPE A																																			
nervous tension																																			
mood swings																																			
irritability																																			
anxiety																																			
TYPE C																																			
headache																																			
craving for sweets																																			
increased appetite																																			
pounding heart																																			
fatigue																																			
tremulousness																																			
TYPE D																																			
depression																																			
forgetfulness																																			
crying																																			
sleeplessness																																			
TYPE H																																			
weight gain																																			
swelling of extremities																																			
breast tenderness																																			
abdominal bloating																																			
DYSMENORRHEA																																			
cramps (low abdominal)																																			
backache																																			
general aches and pains																																			
nausea and vomiting																																			
ACNE																																			
oily skin																																			
oily hair																																			
pimples																																			

MONTHLY CALENDAR OF MENSTRUAL SYMPTOMS

Grade your symptoms as you experience them each month:

☐ None   ⊡ Mild   ◪ Moderate   ■ Severe

DAY OF CYCLE   1 2 3 4 5 6 7 8 9 10 11 12 13 14 15 16 17 18 19 20 21 22 23 24 25 26 27 28 29 30 31 32 33 34 35

TYPE A
nervous tension
mood swings
irritability
anxiety

TYPE C
headache
craving for sweets
increased appetite
pounding heart
fatigue
tremulousness

TYPE D
depression
forgetfulness
crying
sleeplessness

TYPE H
weight gain
swelling of extremities
breast tenderness
abdominal bloating

DYSMENORRHEA
cramps (low abdominal)
backache
general aches and pains
nausea and vomiting

ACNE
oily skin
oily hair
pimples

EATING HABITS AND PMS

Check off the number of times you eat the following foods.

Foods	Never	Once a Month	Once a Week	Twice a Week or More
coffee				
black tea				
soft drinks				
cow's milk				
cow's cheese				
butter				
yogurt				
eggs				
chocolate				
sugar				
alcohol				
beef				
pork				
lamb				
white bread				
white noodles				
white rice				
white-flour pastries				
added salt				
bouillon				
commercial salad dressing				
catsup				
hot dogs				
oranges				
papaya				
pineapple				
tomatoes				

Foods	Never	Once a Month	Once a Week	Twice a Week or More
potatoes				
eggplant				
avocado				
spinach				
beans				
beets				
broccoli				
brussels sprouts				
cabbage				
carrots				
celery				
collard				
cucumbers				
garlic				
horseradish				
kale				
lettuce				
mustard greens				
okra				
onions				
parsnips				
peas				
radishes				
rutabagas				
squash				
turnips				
turnip greens				
yams				

Foods	Never	Once a Month	Once a Week	Twice a Week or More
brown rice				
millet				
oatmeal				
buckwheat				
barley				
rye				
wheat				
corn				
sesame seeds				
sunflower seeds				
pumpkin seeds				
almonds				
peanuts				
apples				
berries				
pears				
seasonal fruits				
corn oil				
olive oil				
sesame oil				
safflower oil				
poultry				
fish				

Key to Eating Habits and Your PMS. All the foods in the shaded area are high-stress foods that can worsen your symptoms of PMS. If you eat a significant number of these foods, or if you eat any of these foods frequently, your nutritional habits may be contributing significantly to your symptoms, and you can probably be helped by Chapters Five through Ten.

All the foods from beans to fish are high-nutrient, low-stress foods that may help to relieve or prevent PMS symptoms and should be included frequently in your diet. If you are already eating many of these foods and few of the high-stress foods, chances are your nutritional habits are good, and nutrition may not be a significant factor in your PMS. Stress-reduction and the exercises and other body work methods beginning on page 143 may be more important to you.

EXERCISE HABITS AND PMS

Check off the number of times you do any of the following.

Exercise	Never	Once a Month	Once or Twice a Week	Three Times a Week or More
fast walking				
running				
swimming				
bicycling				
tennis				
aerobic dancing				
yoga				
other exercise				

Key to Exercise Habits and PMS. Exercise is a good outlet for stress and can improve oxygenation and reduce pain. If your total number of exercise periods per week is less than three, you will probably be more prone to multiple PMS symptoms, and the chapters on various kinds of exercise for PMS will be important to you.

If you are exercising more than three times a week, keep doing your exercises; they are probably making your symptoms less severe. You may want to add specific corrective exercises to your present regime, choosing them to fit your individual symptoms from the chart on page 60.

WHAT STRESS DOES TO YOUR BODY

Check the places where tension most commonly localizes in your body.

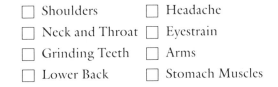

☐ Shoulders   ☐ Headache
☐ Neck and Throat   ☐ Eyestrain
☐ Grinding Teeth   ☐ Arms
☐ Lower Back   ☐ Stomach Muscles

Key to What Stress Does to Your Body. This evaluation should help you become aware of where you sequester stress in your body. Everyone has her own favorite area: tensions automatically accumulate there, like nuts in a squirrel's cheek. This accumulation increases your general level of fatigue and lowers your energy. Storing tension in the spine can worsen cramps; storing it in the neck can cause headaches.

Try to remain aware of the areas where you store tension. When you feel tension building up in them, begin deep breathing. Often this will release the tension immediately. If it does not, use one of the other methods given in the chapter on stress reduction.

MAJOR STRESS EVALUATION

Item Value	Your Score	Life Events
100	_____	Death of spouse
73	_____	Divorce from spouse
65	_____	Separation from spouse
63	_____	Death of a close family member
53	_____	Personal injury or illness (serious)
50	_____	Embark on a new marriage
47	_____	Fired from your steady job
45	_____	Have a marriage reconciliation
45	_____	Enter into retirement from work
44	_____	Change in health of a family member
40	_____	Learn that you are pregnant
39	_____	Difficulties with your sexual abilities
39	_____	Gain a new family member
39	_____	Have a readjustment (major) in business
38	_____	Have a radical change in finances
37	_____	Death of a close relative
36	_____	Change to a different line of work
35	_____	Increase in number of marital arguments
31	_____	Take on a loan or mortgage of more than $70,000
30	_____	Foreclosure of mortgage or loan
29	_____	Responsibilities change at work
29	_____	Son or daughter leaving home
29	_____	Irritating trouble with in-laws
28	_____	Recognition for outstanding achievements
26	_____	Spouse begins or stops work
26	_____	You begin or end schooling
25	_____	You undergo a change in living conditions
24	_____	You revise your personal habits
23	_____	You experience trouble with your boss

This evaluation has been modified from the Life Change Index developed by Dr. Thomas Holmes and his co-workers at the University of Washington Medical School.

Item Value	Your Score	Life Events
20	_____	Work hours or conditions are different
20	_____	You change your residence
20	_____	You change your school or major subject
19	_____	Alterations in your recreation are marked
19	_____	Church or club activities change
18	_____	Social activities change
17	_____	Take on a loan or mortgage of less than $70,000
16	_____	Your sleeping habits change
15	_____	The number of family get-togethers changes
15	_____	Eating habits are altered
13	_____	You go on vacation
12	_____	The year-end holidays occur
11	_____	You commit a minor violation of the law
_____		TOTAL

Key to Major Stress Evaluation. A score of over 300 points on this evaluation indicates major life stress and vulnerability to serious illness. If you scored over 300, do *everything you can to be good to yourself.* Eat well, following the guidelines in Chapter Four; exercise; and learn the methods for managing stress given in the chapter on stress reduction.

If you scored between 200 and 299, you are also at some risk of illness and should follow the suggestions above.

If you scored below 200, you are believed to be at low risk of illness caused by stress. But since stresses too small to figure in this evaluation may also play a part in your PMS, and since it is impossible to predict or prevent the occurrence of certain major stresses, it would still be helpful for you to learn the methods outlined in the chapter on stress reduction.

DAILY STRESS EVALUATION

Check each item that seems to apply to you.

WORK

☐ **Pushing too hard.** Too much responsibility is heaped on you or you push yourself too hard. You worry about getting it all done and doing it well.

☐ **Understimulation.** Work is boring. The lack of stimulation makes you tired. You wish you were somewhere else.

☐ **Time pressure.** You worry about getting your work done on time. You always feel rushed.

☐ **Boss pressure.** Your boss demands too much. Your boss is too picky.

☐ **Uncomfortable physical plant.** Lights are too bright or too dim; noises are too loud. You are exposed to noxious fumes or chemicals. There is too much activity going on around you, making it difficult to concentrate.

HUSBAND OR SIGNIFICANT OTHER

☐ **Communication.** Not enough discussion of feelings. You both tend to hold in emotion. Too much negative emotion and drama. You are always upset and angry. Not enough peace and quiet.

☐ **Discrepancy in communication.** One person talks about feelings too much, the other person too little.

☐ **Affection.** You do not feel that you receive enough affection. There is not enough holding, touching and loving in your relationship. You are made uncomfortable by your partner's demands.

☐ **Sexuality.** Not enough sexual intimacy. You feel deprived by your partner. There is a demand for too-frequent sexual relations by your partner. You feel pressured.

☐ **Children.** They make too much noise. They make too many demands on your time.

☐ **Organization.** Home is poorly organized. It always seems messy, chores are half-finished.

☐ **Time.** Too much to do, never enough time to get it all done.

☐ **Responsibility.** You need more help. Too many demands on your time and energy.

THE INNER YOU

- [ ] **Too much anxiety.** You worry too much about every little thing. You constantly worry about what can go wrong.
- [ ] **Victimization.** Everyone is taking advantage of you or wants to hurt you.
- [ ] **Poor self-image.** You don't like yourself enough. You are always finding fault with yourself.
- [ ] **Too critical.** You are always finding fault with others.
- [ ] **Inability to relax.** You are always wound up. It is difficult for you to relax.
- [ ] **Not enough self-renewal.** You don't play enough or take enough time off to relax and have fun.
- [ ] **Insufficient sleep.** You don't get enough sleep and often feel tired.

Key to Daily Stress Evaluation. This evaluation is included to help you become aware of the minor daily stresses in your life. Although these stresses are not as significant individually as major life stresses and are more difficult to quantify scientifically, they can build up and add significantly to your PMS and other health problems. Becoming aware of them is the first step toward lessening their effects on your life. Methods for reducing them and helping your body to deal with them are given in the chapter on stress reduction.

Part Three:
Finding the Solution

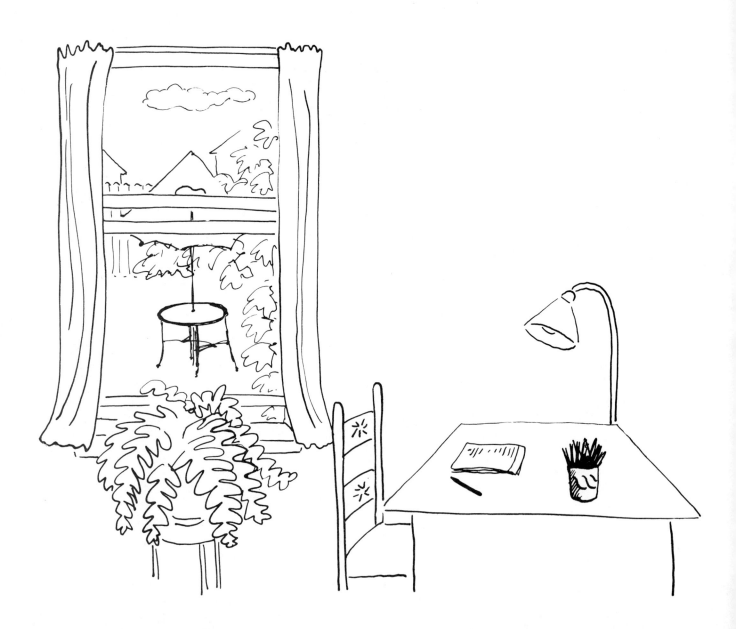

4

The Premenstrual Syndrome Program

Now that you know all about the problem, you are ready to begin your treatment program. This program is set up so that you can individualize a treatment plan for yourself. The methods that you need are contained in the chapters that follow. These include nutrition, stress reduction, exercise, acupressure massage, chiropractic exercises, and yoga.

This chapter contains a master plan that will help you to put your own program together. The chart on the next pages will tell you which treatments to use for your symptoms.

There are two basic ways to use the treatment plan. You can find your symptoms in the chart and turn directly to the treatments for those symptoms. What will work for you can be found easily if you try all the therapies listed under your symptoms. You will probably find that some make you feel better than others. Establish the regimen that works for you and use it each month. Or you can read straight through the rest of the book, get a general overview of the various approaches, and find those you are interested in trying. You can then use the treatment chart for quick spot work and a large overview. Whichever way you choose, if you follow your own plan faithfully, you will begin to see improvements in your symptoms and your life very quickly—within a month or two.

COMPLETE TREATMENT CHART FOR PMS

	Type A *anxiety* *irritability* *mood swings*	Type C *sugar craving* *fatigue* *headaches*	Type H *weight gain* *bloating* *breast tenderness*
Medication	tranquilizers progesterone	analgesics muscle-relaxants	diuretics
Nutrition	The Women's Diet eliminate caffeine, dairy products, chocolate, alcohol	The Women's Diet eliminate sugar, chocolate, alcohol, tropical fruits	The Women's Diet eliminate salt, dairy products
Vitamins	vitamin and mineral formula, page 85 emphasize B complex, magnesium, inositol	vitamin and mineral formula, page 85 emphasize B complex, magnesium	vitamin and mineral formula, page 85 emphasize B complex, magnesium
Herbs	ginger burdock sarsaparilla	ginger burdock sarsaparilla	ginger burdock sarsaparilla
Exercise	moderate exercise walking, jogging, swim- ming, tennis, bicycling	moderate exercise walking, jogging, swim- ming, tennis, bicycling	moderate exercise walking, jogging, swim- ming, tennis, bicycling
Stress Reduction	PMS stress-reduction exercises	PMS stress-reduction exercises	PMS stress-reduction exercises
Acupressure Massage	acupressure exercise 1*, 2	acupressure exercise 1, 2, 7*	acupressure exercise 1, 2, 4*
Neurolymphatic Massage Points	NL-1	NL-3, -4	NL-1, -2
Neurovascular Holding Points	NV-1, -2	NV-2	
Yoga	Pump, Child's Pose Sponge	Spinal Flex, Bow	Wide Angle Pose, Plow, Sponge

*These exercises are particularly effective.

	Type D *depression* *confusion* *memory loss*	Acne *pimples* *oily skin* *oily hair*	Dysmenorrhea *cramps* *low back pain* *nausea, vomiting*
Medication	antidepressants	antibiotics benzyl peroxide	analgesics antiprostaglandins
Nutrition	The Women's Diet eliminate dairy products	The Women's Diet eliminate dairy products, sugar, chocolate, alcohol, nuts	The Women's Diet eliminate dairy products
Vitamins	vitamin and mineral formula, page 85 emphasize B complex, magnesium	vitamin and mineral formula, page 85 emphasize vitamin A, choline, inositol	vitamin and mineral formula, page 85 magnesium, calcium
Herbs	ginger licorice	burdock dandelion alfalfa	ginger
Exercise	moderate exercise walking, jogging, swim- ming, tennis, bicycling	moderate exercise walking, jogging, swim- ming, tennis, bicycling	moderate exercise walking, jogging, swim- ming, tennis, bicycling
Stress Reduction	PMS stress-reduction exercises	PMS stress-reduction exercises	PMS stress-reduction exercises
Acupressure Massage	acupressure exercise 2, 7*	acupressure exercise 1, 2, 6*	acupressure exercise 1, 2, 3*, 4*, 5*
Neurolymphatic Massage Points	NL-1	NL-2	NL-5
Neurovascular Holding Points	NV-1, -2		
Yoga	Upward-Facing Dog Bow	Spinal Flex, Bow,	Arm and Leg Stretch, Pump, Locust, Plow, Sponge, Bow, Child's Pose

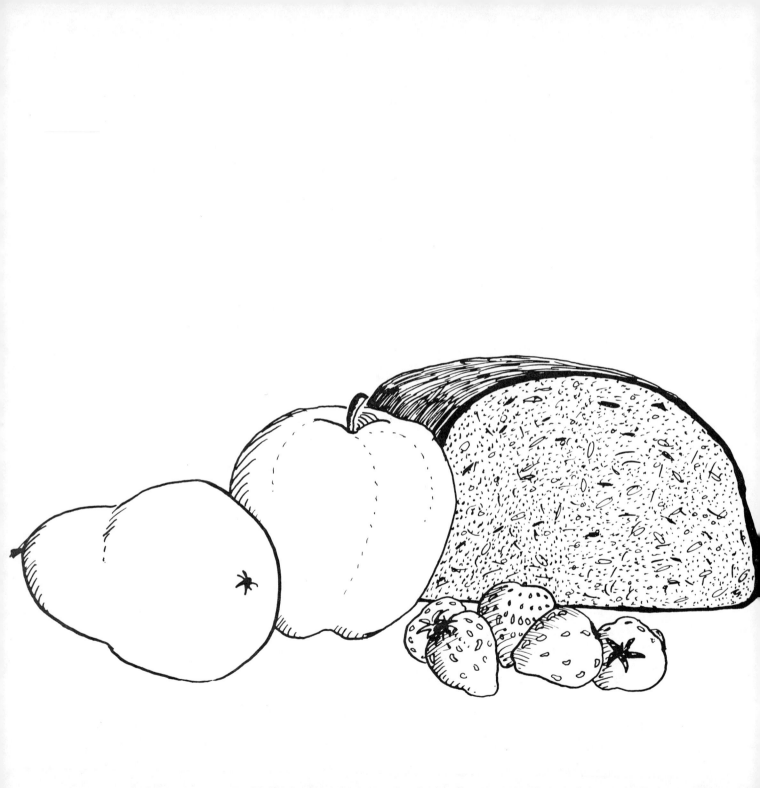

5

The Women's Diet: Nutrition for a Life Free of PMS

It is impossible to overestimate the importance of good nutrition in controlling PMS. No medication can entirely overcome the effects of a poor diet. And no medical cure, however miraculous, can ever be as satisfactory as the changes we see in patients who come to us in desperation, sometimes with such severe physical and mental symptoms that they are at the point of hospitalizing themselves, and are back after several months on our special Women's Diet, not only free of their original symptoms, but also reporting that they have more energy and a greater sense of well-being than they have had in years. (Sometimes they tell us that symptoms they had never associated with their PMS, such as allergies and phobias, have disappeared too.)

I call the diet the Women's Diet rather than the PMS diet because it is more than just the sum of our knowledge about what is bad and what is good for PMS. It is really the diet that every woman above the age of puberty should follow (with small adjustments for pregnancy and menopause) in order to be in the best possible health.

It is shocking at first to see the list of foods that worsen PMS. It includes many staples of the American diet and many of the foods women automatically turn to when they feel tired and want a pick-me-up (or when they feel depressed and seek solace in food). But the fact is that these foods have almost all become important in our diet within the last hundred years. They are not part of our nutritional heritage. Many of them are truly addictive and have the importance they do in our diet because they cause cycles of binging and hunger.

It may take from three months to two years to get completely free of these foods, but once you do, they will exert very little attraction, particularly in comparison to the new foods you will have added to your diet.

Fortunately, the list of foods that are good for PMS is also a long one. And once you learn the knack of preparing them, they are no less sensuous or convenient than the foods that are bad for PMS.

The Women's Diet is not a diet of self-denial. As I think you'll see when you begin cooking from the cookbook (page 115), it does not require sacrifices of either taste or ease of preparation. Many of these meals can be prepared in fifteen to twenty minutes and require only a few ingredients.

There is also no reason to sacrifice amenity or the fun of entertaining. The foods on the Women's Diet are nutritious for the whole family and can be presented as elegantly as anything in classical French cuisine.

The Women's Diet is the result of nine years of experience with PMS patients. Unfortunately, I feel I have to warn against some diets that have been put forth as diets for PMS, but do not seem to be based on clinical experience. Many of them are unsound and unsafe. I particularly hope that you have not been following the diet (recommended in a recent book) that includes orange juice, tomatoes, dairy products, and beef. This is a diet not to cure PMS but to cause it. It runs counter to almost every known nutritional model, including those of PMS expert Dr. Guy Abraham, naturopathic theorists, Japanese macrobiotic practitioners, Chinese nutritionists, and even the American Heart Association.

In the guidelines that follow, the physiology behind the Women's Diet is explained in the terms of Western medicine. It seems worthwhile to mention, though, that the same foods would be indicated by the traditional Oriental health model. This model presents the world as a balance of opposing elements: *yin,* which covers all those body elements, health conditions and foods that are cool, passive, negative, sugar-containing, water-containing, and expansive; and *yang,* which describes those that are hot, active, positive, salt-containing, and contracting. Yin foods include fruits, candies, white flour, and milk products. Yang foods include eggs and meats and salty and pickled foods. Neutral foods include grains, beans, fish, vegetables, sea vegetables, and temperate-climate fruits taken in small amounts. To eat predominantly at either end of the spectrum is considered stressful to the body and likely to predispose to disease. Interestingly enough, extreme yin and extreme yang foods are identical to high-stress foods that may worsen PMS in the Western model.

FOODS THAT WORSEN PMS

The Women's Diet limits, first and foremost:

- Foods that are high in refined sugars and fats.
- Foods that are highly processed and full of chemicals.

These include cola drinks, chocolate, alcohol, candy, ice cream, hamburgers, hot dogs, hard cheese, beef, pork, lamb, and pizza. These foods appeal to the palate and provide quick energy, but most of them provide very few nutrients and can disrupt your hormonal chemistry. If you have PMS, you probably have a craving for one or more of these foods. They can be hard to kick, which is why the more detailed table of PMS-causing foods on page 66 includes foods to substitute as well.

Foods that Worsen PMS (and Reasons Why)	Foods to Substitute
Caffeinated beverages, including *coffee, tea,* and *cola drinks.* Caffeine can cause breast tenderness. Fifteen to 30 percent of women with breast tenderness note relief upon stopping caffeine-containing beverages. Caffeine also increases anxiety, irritability and mood swings and depletes the body's stores of vitamin B—thus interfering with carbohydrate metabolism.	Water-process *decaffeinated coffee* is often the easiest substitute to start with for those women who like the flavor of coffee. Coffee substitutes that are grain-based, such as *Pero, Postum,* and *Caffix,* are even better. *Herbal teas,* such as chamomile and hops, can actually be therapeutic for women with anxiety, since they have a calming and sedative effect.
Dairy products, including *cow's milk, cow's cheese, butter, and yogurt;* and *eggs.* These foods interfere with the absorption of magnesium, a mineral that can decrease cramps, help glucose metabolism, and stabilize mood swings. Their high sodium content can worsen fluid retention and bloating. Their high fat content decreases the liver's efficiency in metabolizing hormones. The tryptophan in cow's-milk products increases fatigue.	Use *smaller amounts of cow's-milk products.* For example, use cheese as a garnish for soups, salads, and casseroles, not as a major source of protein. *Goat's* or *sheep's cheese* can be used to replace cow's cheese, since the fat they contain is more easily emulsified in the body. *Soy milk* and *nut milks* (available at most health food stores) are good sources of calcium and can be used for drinking, eating with cereal or baking. *Vegetable cooking water, rice water,* or *potato water* can be substituted for milk or cream as a thickener for sauces. (Add one cup of cooked rice or a cooked diced potato to half a cup of water and blend in blender.) *Apple juice* can be substituted for milk in baking. As a substitute for whipped cream, mash a *banana,* add the beaten *white of one egg,* and beat until stiff. As a substitute for butter, mix cold-pressed *corn oil* with sea salt. (Herbs

(continued)

Foods that Worsen PMS (and Reasons Why)	Foods to Substitute

can also be added.) Mixture will thicken if refrigerated and can then be spread with spoon or pastry brush. One teaspoon of *baking powder* can be substituted for each egg in a recipe. Baked goods will be flatter, but will still taste good. *Puréed vegetables* or *applesauce* will give body and moisture to baked goods. Good sources of calcium include *green leafy vegetables* (collard, kale, mustard greens), *beans, peas, soybeans, sesame seeds, carob, fish,* and *chicken stock* made with bones.

Chocolate worsens mood swings, intensifies sugar craving, causes weight gain, and increases demand for the B-complex vitamins. It also causes breast tenderness.

Unsweetened carob tastes like chocolate but is far more nutritious (although it, too, is high in calories and fat and should be eaten in small amounts). It is a member of the legume family and is high in calcium. It can be purchased in chunk form as a substitute for chocolate candy or as a powder to be used in baking or drinks. The magnesium chocolate provides can be found in many other foods. (See page 80.)

Sugar depletes the body's B-complex vitamins and minerals and intensifies sugar craving and the symptoms of Type C.

Sweeter foods in smaller measure. Honey is two and a half times as sweet as sugar. *Maple syrup* is also sweeter and more concentrated than sugar. *Apple juice* can also be used as a substitute in baking. (See substitution tables on page 134.)

(continued)

Foods that Worsen PMS (and Reasons Why)	Foods to Substitute
Alcohol depletes the body's vitamin B and minerals, disrupts carbohydrate metabolism, and intensifies symptoms of Type C. Alcohol is toxic to the liver and can disrupt the liver's ability to metabolize hormones, thus causing higher-than-normal estrogen.	*Light wine* and *beer* in small amounts have a lower alcohol content than hard liquor, liqueurs, and regular wine. A nonalcoholic cocktail such as *mineral water* with a twist of lime or lemon or a dash of bitters is an even better substitute. *Near beer*, a nonalcoholic beer substitute, tastes quite a bit like the real thing.
Beef, pork, and *lamb* all have a high fat content that can compromise liver efficiency. Some beef contains small amounts of synthetic estrogens to increase growth of cattle. Too much protein increases demand for minerals.	Substitute *chicken, turkey,* or *fish*. There are also some good vegetable sources of protein, including *whole grains, beans* and *peas, seeds,* and *nuts*. These tend to be versatile foods and contain fiber, complex carbohydrates, and many vitamins and minerals.
Salt and *high-sodium foods* such as bouillon, commercial salad dressings, catsup, and hot dogs all worsen fluid retention, bloating, and breast tenderness.	*Potassium-based salt substitutes are much less harmful. Kelp* is a delicious sea vegetable product. It is also an excellent source of iodine and other trace minerals. *Herbs mixed with a small amount of sea salt* make a delicious condiment.
Oranges, grapefruit, papaya, pineapple, tomatoes, potatoes, eggplant, avocado, and *spinach*. Most of these are higher in simple sugars than other fruits and vegetables. In Oriental medicine, all these foods are considered extremely "yin," thus bad for PMS.	*Other fruits and vegetables.*

FOODS THAT HELP PMS

The Women's Diet emphasizes the use of whole fresh foods. It is a return to the diet to which our bodies adapted over thousands of years. It emphasizes:

Foods Made from Whole Grains

Whole Grains. Whole grains (including wheat, corn, barley, oats, rye, millet, buckwheat and brown rice) are complex carbohydrates, capable of stabilizing your blood sugar and helping tremendously to eliminate premenstrual sugar craving. They contain excellent sources of protein, fiber, vitamins B and E, and various minerals. They can be prepared in a variety of ways.

Whole-grain Cereals. Whole-grain cereals, either hot or cold, will help your PMS. Your best bets if you shop in a local supermarket are Wheatina, Maltex, or the *slow-cooking* Quaker's Oats (the quick-cooking kind is a refined grain product and should be avoided if you have PMS). Health food stores offer a larger choice of cereals. Puffed millet, puffed corn, and puffed rice are all available as cold breakfast cereals. Unsweetened granola, cream of rye and buckwheat groats are also good.

Whole-grain Bread. Take advantage of the many different whole-grain breads that are available at health food stores today—rice, sesame-millet, oatmeal, soy-potato, rye, and lima bean bread, among others. Choose brands without added sugar.

Crackers. Crackers can be used for snacks or open-faced sandwiches. Brown rice cakes are a particularly good snack.

Spread with nut butters or fruit preserves, they help stabilize the blood sugar level in women with Type C.

Pancakes and Waffles. Pancakes and waffles can be made with whole wheat, buckwheat, or rice flour. Concentrated forms of sweeteners such as maple syrup, honey, and applesauce can be used in small amounts.

Pasta. When the word pasta is mentioned, most women think of refined wheat noodles and spaghetti, but buckwheat, rice, corn, soy, and whole wheat pastas are also available— and much more nutritious. Whole grain pasta is also made with several delicately flavored vegetables, including artichokes and spinach.

Legumes

Lentils, kidney beans, pinto beans, mung beans, garbanzo beans, adzuki beans, green peas, and the many other members of the legume family can be used in many ways. They can become bases for thick soups. They can be eaten in salads or used in dips and casseroles. When eaten with grains they form a complete protein comparable to that in eggs or meat.

Seeds and Nuts

Seeds and nuts are excellent sources of protein. They should be either dry-roasted or raw and unsalted. They are very high in calories so quantities consumed should be moderate if premenstrual weight gain is a problem for you. If you have acne, eat only very small amounts.

Vegetables

Most vegetables are rich in vitamins and minerals. Particularly good for women with PMS are root vegetables such as rutabagas, carrots, turnips, and parsnips and the leafy green vegetables such as kale, collard, and mustard greens. There are very few (spinach, avocados, potatoes, tomatoes, and eggplant) that intensify PMS.

Fruits

The best fruits for PMS are those that are seasonal and grown in temperate climates. They tend to be higher in fiber and lower in sugar content. Fruits grown in the hot tropical sun tend to be much sweeter, which can worsen fluid retention and sugar craving in susceptible women.

Oils

Preferred oils include sesame oil, olive oil, corn oil, and safflower oil. Unlike animal fats, they are unsaturated. (All except olive oil are polyunsaturated.) Cold-pressed oils tend to be fresher and purer.

Foods from Other Cultures That Can Help PMS

Excellent foods from other cultures are available in health food stores and ethnic markets, especially Oriental markets. Many of them are very useful for women with PMS. High-nutrient condiments are available that can be used to flavor your foods. Some are prized in their countries of origin for their medicinal value and for their ability to balance the body chemistry. Japanese women who eat the traditional diet of grains, fermented bean products, and sea vegetables have much less tendency toward diseases due to hormonal imbalance (such as PMS, breast cancer, and fibroid tumors) than American women on a high-fat, high-sugar diet. You might want to try these foods in small amounts. If you enjoy their flavors, they would be beneficial additions to your diet.

Miso. Miso is a high-nutrient fermented soy product. It is very helpful in fighting fatigue and in combating the morning blahs. It is an excellent source of complete protein, since it contains all eight essential amino acids. It contains between 12 and 20 percent protein (compared to 21 percent for chicken, 20 percent for beef, 13 percent for eggs and 3 percent for whole cow's milk). It is also a good source of minerals such as calcium and iron.

Miso aids in the digestion and assimilation of other foods, since it is high in both digestive enzymes and acidophilus bacteria. It is also a useful source of vitamin B_{12} for women on a vegetarian diet.

Miso is a good salt substitute. (One-half teaspoon of miso is the equivalent of one tablespoon of salt.) It can be used in soups, salad dressings, dips, and spreads for crackers. (See "The Women's Diet Cookbook," beginning on page 115.)

Tamari Soy Sauce. Tamari soy sauce is another fermented soy product (made from water, salt and soybeans). It is used to give flavor when stir-frying foods. It can be used in small amounts as a salt substitute. One-quarter teaspoon of tamari soy sauce has the seasoning power of one teaspoon of salt, and contains much less sodium. (A teaspoon of salt has approximately 2,000 milligrams of sodium. By comparison, a teaspoon of tamari has only about 270 milligrams.)

Kelp. This is a powdered seaweed product. It contains several dozen minerals. It is high in iodine, which is critical for normal thyroid function. Kelp can also be used as a salt substitute. It can be kept in a salt shaker and added to food at the table. It is delicious when added to soups and casseroles.

Gomasio. Gomasio is a third alternative to table salt. It consists of sea salt added to ground and toasted sesame seeds. Sesame seeds are high in protein, calcium, iron, and phosphorus.

Umeboshi Plums. These pickled plums are used in teas, soups, and salad dressings. They are used in Oriental healing to maintain acid-alkaline balance. They are sharp-tasting and can cause the mouth to pucker if eaten by themselves. An excellent tea recipe is as follows:

> 1 umeboshi plum
> 1 teaspoon kudzu herb
> 1 teaspoon grated ginger

Add to 1 pint of water, boil, and steep. Upon serving, add a few drops of tamari. The remaining tea can be refrigerated and used later. This tea is excellent in the morning for women with premenstrual fatigue. The ingredients may be purchased at well-stocked health food stores and Oriental markets.

SHOPPING LIST FOR PMS

Vegetables

beans
beets
broccoli
brussels sprouts
cabbage
carrots
celery
collard
cucumbers
garlic
horseradish
kale
lettuce
mustard greens
okra
onions
parsnips
peas
radishes
rutabagas
squash
turnips
turnip greens
yams

Whole Grains

brown rice
millet
oatmeal
buckwheat
barley
rye
wheat (unless you
   are allergic to it)
corn

Seeds and Nuts

sesame seeds
sunflower seeds
pumpkin seeds
almonds
   (or walnuts, pecans,
   cashews, or filberts)
peanuts

Fruits

apples
berries
pears
seasonal fruits
   (one per day)

Oils

corn
olive
sesame
safflower

Foods from Other Cultures

miso
tamari soy sauce
kelp
gomasio
umeboshi plums

Meats

poultry
fish
seafood
   (in moderation)

6

Vitamins and Minerals for PMS

There are a number of vitamins and minerals that are important in overcoming PMS. If you shop from the PMS shopping list on page 74, eat a variety of foods and rotate those foods, you will get most of what you need. But if you have a particularly stubborn symptom, you may want to emphasize the foods (and vitamin supplements) that are high in the elements that help it. (For example, a woman with acne might want to eat more carrots; a woman with cramps more leafy green vegetables; a woman with heavy bleeding more beet greens.)

The Vitamins and Minerals and What They Do

Vitamin A. Vitamin A helps to improve the health of your skin. It is useful in suppressing premenstrual acne and oily skin. There are two types of vitamin A. Vitamin A from animal sources such as fish oil is stored in the liver and can be toxic if taken in too large a dose (greater than 40,000 international units [I.U.] a day for several months). Carotene, a precursor of vitamin A found in plant sources, is more easily

Adult recommended daily allowance: 5,000 I.U.

Therapeutic requirements for PMS: 15,000 to 40,000 I.U.

carrots
butternut squash
salmon
dandelion greens
Hubbard squash
sweet potatoes
turnip greens
kale
mustard greens
beet greens
bok choy
broccoli
sweet red peppers
apricots
romaine lettuce
peaches
asparagus
butter lettuce

absorbed upon ingestion. It is not toxic in large amounts. A single carrot can have as much as 10,000 I.U. Some other good food sources of vitamin A are listed at left.

Vitamin-B Complex. The vitamin-B complex consists of eleven factors that work together to perform important metabolic functions, including glucose metabolism, inactivation of estrogen by the liver, and stabilization of brain chemistry. The B-complex vitamins are usually found together in foods such as whole grains, brewer's yeast, liver, and legumes, but the relative amounts of the individual factors vary considerably from food to food.

Emotional stress causes loss of the water-soluble B vitamins from the body. Fatigue and irritability can be the result.

My recommended therapeutic dosages for PMS (PMS-RDA) for some of the important B vitamins are:

	PMS-RDA
Thiamine (vitamin B_1)	50 mg.
Riboflavin (vitamin B_2)	50 mg.
Niacin (vitamin B_3)	50 mg.
Biotin	30 mcg.
Pantothenic acid (vitamin B_5)	50 mg.
Pyridoxine (vitamin B_6)	300 mg.
Para-aminobenzoic acid	50 mg.
Choline	500 mg.
Inositol	500 mg.
Cyanocobalamin (vitamin B_{12})	50 mcg.
Folic acid	200 mcg.

Choline and Inositol. Among the B vitamins, choline, inositol and B_6 are known to be of particular importance in preventing PMS. Choline and inositol enhance the liver's ability to break down fatty foods and fat-soluble hormones such as estrogen. Inositol is also a central nervous system tranquilizer and may help to calm premenstrual anxiety and irritability. Inositol and choline are found in high amounts in soybeans, wheat germ, bran and corn.

Vitamin B_6. Vitamin B_6, in doses up to 300 milligrams, can help to regulate many premenstrual symptoms, including mood swings, irritability, fluid retention, breast tenderness, bloating, sugar craving, and fatigue. Vitamin B_6 levels decrease in women using birth control pills. Food sources of vitamin B_6 are listed on this page.

If you take individual B vitamins, it's important to take the rest of the complex, too.

SOME FOOD SOURCES OF VITAMIN B_6
(in order, from best to good)

Adult recommended daily allowance: 2 milligrams

Therapeutic requirements for PMS: 300 milligrams

salmon	rye flour
chicken	brown rice
tuna	broccoli
soybeans	asparagus
rice bran	wheat germ
rice polishings	brussels sprouts
kale	torula yeast
buckwheat flour	beet greens
navy beans	green peas
lentils	sunflower seeds
lima beans	sweet potatoes
pinto beans	cauliflower
black-eyed peas	brewer's yeast
shrimp	leeks
whole wheat flour	

Vitamin C. Vitamin C is an important antioxidant and anti-stress vitamin. It is necessary for adrenal cortical hormone synthesis and for immune function. It also has an antihistamine effect, which can help women whose allergies worsen before their periods.

SOME FOOD SOURCES OF VITAMIN C
(in order, from best to good)

Adult recommended daily allowance: 45 milligrams

Therapeutic requirements for PMS: 500 milligrams to 3 grams

sweet red peppers	lemons
brussels sprouts	turnips
collard greens	peas
sorrel	red raspberries
kale	blackberries
green peppers	lima beans
strawberries	chard leaves
lamb's-quarters	tomatoes
kohlrabi	spinach
cauliflower	pineapples
mustard greens	sweet potatoes
oranges	potatoes
grapefruit	blueberries
cabbage	mung bean sprouts
rutabagas	bananas
salmon	chicken
lemons	

SOME FOOD SOURCES OF VITAMIN E
(in order, from best to good)

Adult recommended daily allowance: 12 to 15 I.U.

Therapeutic requirements for PMS: 400 to 800 I.U.

wheat germ oil
walnut oil
sunflower oil
sweet potatoes
safflower oil
turnip greens
beet greens
leeks
wheat germ
asparagus
corn oil
sesame oil
peanut oil
broccoli
brussels sprouts
apples
rye
peas
corn
parsnips
blackberries
cornmeal
wheat

Vitamin D. Vitamin D is essential for the absorption of calcium from the intestinal tract. It can also decrease the skin oiliness that exacerbates premenstrual acne. It is commonly derived either from exposure to the sun or from supplements added to foods, primarily dairy products, sold commercially. Vitamin D is a fat-soluble vitamin that is stored in the liver. Because it tends to accumulate in the body and can cause hazardous side effects in large amounts, vitamin D should not be taken in large doses. It should be taken in soluble form.

Vitamin E. Vitamin E is an important antioxidant. It protects the cells from the destructive effects of many environmental chemicals that can react with the polyunsaturated fats in the cell membranes. Oxidation of the cell can accelerate the aging process as well as many diseases. Early research linked adequate levels of vitamin E with fertility in rats. This suggested that vitamin E has a powerful effect on the hormonal system. This has been corroborated in the last ten years by the work done on fibrocystic breast disease and vitamin E. Up to one half of women with fibrocystic breast changes had resolution of their cysts when using 600 I.U. of vitamin E per day.

Calcium. Calcium helps maintain normal muscle tone and helps prevent cramps and pain. It is present in the foods listed on page 80.

Magnesium. Magnesium is needed to decrease menstrual cramps and control premenstrual sugar craving. It helps to normalize glucose metabolism and stabilize moods by its effect on brain chemistry. Magnesium actually optimizes the amount of usable calcium in your system by increasing calcium absorption. Conversely, calcium can interfere with

SOME FOOD SOURCES OF CALCIUM
(in order, from best to good)

Adult recommended daily allowance: 800 milligrams Therapeutic requirements for PMS: 800 milligrams

- collard leaves
- salmon
- shrimp
- blackstrap molasses
- sesame seeds
- bok choy
- kale
- mustard greens
- broccoli
- tofu
- okra
- dandelion greens
- masa harina
- soybeans
- carob flour
- rutabagas

SOME FOOD SOURCES OF MAGNESIUM
(in order, from best to good)

Adult recommended daily allowance: 350 milligrams

Therapeutic requirements for PMS: 300 milligrams (in supplement)

- soybeans
- beet greens
- black-eyed peas
- shrimp
- white beans
- limas
- red beans
- buckwheat
- salmon
- whole wheat flour
- tofu
- turnip greens
- collards
- cornmeal
- wheat berries
- millet
- dandelion greens
- chicken
- lentils
- cashews
- rye flour
- mustard greens
- brown rice
- peas
- oatmeal
- sweet potatoes
- brussels sprouts
- kale
- almonds
- snap beans
- sesame seeds
- parsnips
- peanut butter
- filberts (hazelnuts)
- beets
- turnips
- corn
- broccoli
- cauliflower
- pistachios
- whole wheat bread
- barley
- pecans
- summer squash
- onions
- asparagus
- peanuts
- carrots
- tomatoes
- walnuts
- green peppers
- mushrooms
- celery
- cabbage
- sunflower seeds
- lettuce

magnesium absorption. It is usually recommended that the diet include twice as much calcium as magnesium, but for the PMS patient, the ratio should be reversed. Food sources of magnesium are listed on page 80.

Zinc. Zinc is important in conjunction with vitamin A and C for the healing of wounds and the control of acne. It competes with copper for binding sites and displaces copper in the body. Thus an adequate dietary supply of zinc is important

SOME FOOD SOURCES OF ZINC
(in order, from best to good)

Adult recommended daily allowance: 15 milligrams

Therapeutic requirements for PMS: 15 to 25 milligrams

soy meal	millet
wheat bran	soy protein
wheat germ	apples
chicken	corn
rice bran	cabbage
black-eyed peas	onions
whole wheat flour	whole wheat bread
wheat berries	peanut butter
green peas	margarine
cornmeal	carrots
garbanzos	rye bread
lentils	lettuce
limas	snap green beans
soy flour	salad or cooking oil
buckwheat	applesauce
oatmeal	peaches
brown rice	barley

because an overabundance of copper can increase moodiness and increase levels of estrogen. Much of the world's soil is zinc-depleted so it has become more difficult to obtain enough zinc in the diet.

Vitamin and Mineral Supplements for Women with PMS

Good dietary habits are crucial for control of your PMS. But for many women, the use of a nutritional supplement is important in order to achieve high levels of certain essential nutrients. I have formulated a vitamin-and-mineral supplement based on a review of forty years of medical research in this field. This supplement is unlike most of those that are commercially available because the levels of nutrients are specific for the treatment of PMS. I have found it to be very helpful to my patients. This supplement is available by mail order (page 232) or you can put it together yourself. The ingredients are listed at the end of this section in their exact amounts.

If you are like most women, you can take smaller doses during the time when you are symptom-free. If you use my own formulation, two to three pills may be enough to help keep you in optimal health. During the second half of the cycle when your symptoms occur, double the dose. If you know very accurately when your symptoms will begin, you might increase the dose of the supplement a few days ahead. Do not exceed six to eight tablets without the supervision of your physician.

Herbs That Help PMS

Herbs, the traditional treatment for illness for thousands of years, were originally tested not by modern methods but empirically, as people tried them and noted their effects. The body of knowledge thus acquired is still available to us today, and many of my patients prefer plant-based remedies to the drugs offered by modern pharmacology.

Herbs can be looked upon as a form of extended nutrition. Since they are plants, they can make up part of your regular diet when used in small amounts. They help to balance the body chemistry and correct disease symptoms due to nutritional factors. For example, cold symptoms can occur when people eat an abundance of high-stress foods. Medicinal herbs such as burdock and kudzu plus a light diet of vegetables and whole grains can help to correct the imbalance and relieve the cold symptoms. If you are under stress and feel anxious, herbs such as valerian and chamomile can help to stabilize your mood because they calm and tranquilize the central nervous system. Herbs that have been used traditionally to relieve hormonal problems in women include black cohosh, licorice, blessed thistle, damiana, sarsaparilla, red raspberry leaf, wild yam, and gotu kola. For decades, herbalists have observed that these herbs have effects similar to female hormones.

I use herbs in my medical practice as a means of balancing the diet and optimizing the nutritional intake. For example, in Oriental medicine, acne is thought to be due to a predominantly yin or expansive diet that is high in sugar and fat. This can be corrected by balancing the diet with herbs such as dandelion root or burdock root, which are bitter and highly concentrated in their mineral content. In contrast, menstrual cramps are thought to be due to an excess of yang foods such as meat and salt. These are foods that have a contracting effect on the body. For some women, this can be countered by chewing a yin root like ginger, which causes dilation of the blood vessels and relaxation.

Some herbs contain high concentrations of nutrients such as calcium, magnesium, and potassium, which Western medical research has found to be important in controlling a variety of PMS symptoms.

I have found two herbal formulas to be helpful for women suffering from PMS. One formula can be used by women who suffer from any of the following symptoms: mood swings, irritability, anxiety, sugar craving, shakiness, bloating, breast tenderness, and weight gain. This formula contains burdock root, ginger root, and sarsaparilla. A second formula can be used by women with acne and oily skin. This formula contains dandelion, alfalfa, and burdock root. These can be ordered by mail through the PMS Self-Help Center. (See page 232.)

The herbs should be used in small amounts and taken with your meals either in capsule form or in a tea. If you prefer to make a tea, simply empty the capsule into a cup of boiling water and let it steep for a few minutes. Do not drink more than one or two cups of the tea per day. There are some contraindications to the use of herbs. Herbs should not be used if you are currently on a hormone prescribed for you by your doctor.

All foods have the potential for causing distress in some people. Herbs are no exception. They should be discontinued immediately if you notice nausea, vomiting, or diarrhea upon using. These are the most common symptoms of intolerance. The herbs in my formula are all recommended as being safe for human consumption, but some women seem to have a specific intolerance for various foods, including herbs. If you notice *any* symptoms that make you uncomfortable after using the herbs, discontinue them immediately.

OPTIMAL NUTRITIONAL SUPPLEMENTATION FOR PMS

Vitamins

Beta carotene	15,000 I.U.
Vitamin B_1 (thiamine)	50 mg.
Vitamin B_2	50 mg.
Niacinamide	50 mg.
Pantothenic acid	50 mg.
Vitamin B_6 (pyridoxine HCl)	300 mg.
Folic acid	200 mcg.
Biotin	30 mcg.
Vitamin B_{12}	50 mcg.
Choline bitartrate	500 mg.
Inositol	500 mg.
PABA (para-aminobenzoic acid)	50 mg.
Vitamin C	1,000 mg.
Vitamin D (cholecalciferol)	100 I.U.
Vitamin E	600 I.U.

Minerals

Calcium (amino acid chelate)	150mg.
Magnesium	300 mg.
Iodine	150 mcg.
Iron (amino acid chelate)	15 mg.
Copper	0.5 mg.
Zinc	25 mg.
Manganese	10 mg.
Potassium	100 mg.
Selenium	25 mcg.
Chromium	100 mcg.

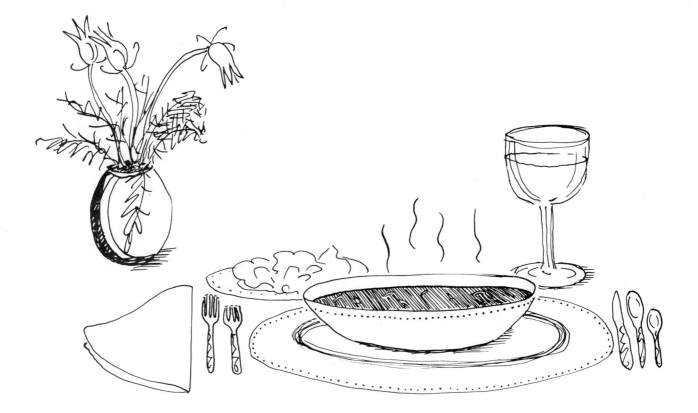

7

Principles of the Women's Diet

Your Diet Should Provide the Greatest Possible Variety

Rotate your foods. This minimizes symptoms of food allergy, which can be worse before your period. It also guarantees that you will be taking in a larger range of nutrients. Many women fall into the rut of eating the same foods day after day. They will go to the same shelves of the supermarket out of habit and convenience. There is safety in familiarity, sticking with a tried formula even if it adversely affects your health in the long run. Also, it takes time to learn new cooking methods. In this chapter and in Chapter Nine, I have provided some very simple guidelines and shortcuts for food preparation that should help you get past the initial fear of trying a greater variety of foods.

Foods Should Be Simple and Easy to Prepare

Women today live very complex lives. Many have the responsibility of running households and holding full-time jobs. This does not leave much time for meal-planning and cooking. It is no wonder so many women turn to convenience foods. Fortunately, nutritious foods can be just as convenient as less nutritious foods. Over the years, my patients and I have worked out many shortcuts for preparing high-quality food. Many of them have used these shortcuts to great advantage, and can prepare a complete meal in fifteen to twenty minutes. These shortcuts are given in Chapters Nine and Eleven so that you can use them, too.

Nutritional Changes Should Be Fun

The suggestions in this book offer a chance to taste new types of food and try out new recipes. Approach tasting new foods as you would going to a new restaurant—with a sense of excitement. Many people consider dietary changes a punishment and think that once their symptoms of PMS are better, they can go back to their old eating habits. But it is these habits that caused PMS in the first place, and they are something to be left behind.

To maximize your enjoyment of your new diet, emphasize the aesthetics of dining. A tablecloth, candles and attractive serving dishes can dress up even simple fare. Highlight the color and texture of each food by using side dishes for serving. Try to serve foods with complementary colors. You will be widening your choice of nutrients as well as increasing the eye appeal. (For example, red and yellow vegetables are high in vitamin A, while green vegetables are higher in vitamin C.) This attention to dining aesthetics will increase your emotional gratification and sense of well-being.

Meals Can Still Be Family Affairs

Eating to relieve PMS doesn't mean that you have to sit in a corner and eat by yourself. The nutritional suggestions made in this book can be used with benefit by all members of your family and friends. Most of my patients find that their families enjoy sharing the new foods, as well as feeling healthier. Most dishes can be easily adapted to everyone's taste. If your children insist that life is empty without cheese or hamburger, add extra cheese and hamburger to one side of a casserole. Or prepare your side of a dish without the rich gravy that the rest of your family likes, or add more vegetables.

Chew Your Food Thoroughly

This is particularly important during the healing phase of PMS when you are trying to relieve the body of all significant stress. The first stage of digestion occurs in the mouth. Slow, thorough eating allows the food to be broken down before it reaches the stomach. Eating fast puts a strain on your digestive system. It will also cause you to eat more because you do not feel satiated until twenty minutes after you start eating. This can be a particular problem if weight gain or bloating are among your symptoms.

Eating high-stress foods like beef, dairy products, and sugary products can cause fatigue or a sensation of heaviness. The tiredness that so many women with PMS complain about can be exacerbated by these foods because so much energy is involved in the digestive process.

Eat Heavier Meals Early in the Day, Lighter Meals in the Evening

Digesting food while you are asleep puts a large metabolic load on your entire system. The night is the time when your body repairs itself. It is unhealthy during this rest period to ask your body to continue to work.

Changes Can Be Made Slowly

I have found in my medical practice that it takes anywhere from a month to two years to change one's dietary habits so that these changes feel comfortable and pleasurable (not just healthy). It is unrealistic to expect that you will throw away every high-stress food in your cupboard because you have PMS.

Look back at the list in Chapter Five of foods that worsen PMS. Pick one or two foods from this list that you would be willing to give up immediately. Then look at the list of foods to substitute. For example, if you drink six cups of coffee a day and start your morning with orange juice, you might decide to switch to a coffee substitute like Pero and substitute a small piece of apple for the orange juice. You may not want to make any other changes until a month later. When you are comfortable with these changes, go back to your list of foods to limit. Perhaps now you are ready to cut down on your intake of dairy products. Perhaps you could eliminate the slice of cheese from your sandwich at lunch. Instead of yogurt, you might take a bowl of soup.

Every few weeks go back to the list of foods to limit and foods to emphasize. Pick a few more foods to eliminate and a few more foods to add to your diet. Remember that *even modest dietary changes can bring significant relief of your PMS.* On the other hand, some people find it easier to change their diets by giving up foods abruptly, and that is fine too. The important thing is to find the way that will work for you.

8

How to Beat the Most Common Eating Problems for Women

Food addictions like sugar craving, caffeine dependency, and eating binges may not sound serious in comparison to more socially proscribed addictions, but they cause a lot of trouble in women's lives and are difficult to overcome. They can be beaten, however, as my patients and I have discovered.

How to Cut Sugar Craving

Breaking the cycle of addiction to sugar is not easy. It is a particularly acute problem for women who have intellectually demanding jobs or hobbies (for example, reading or writing). The brain is a major user of the available sugar in the blood: after intense mental activity, the blood sugar level drops and the brain signals for more glucose. During the premenstrual period, the demand for sugar becomes even stronger.

Most women respond to the demand for sugar by going for quick energy sources such as fruit juice, chocolate, candy, cake, or cookies—anything sweet that's around the house. This works for the short term, but in the long run it causes an erratic, roller-coaster pattern in which the pancreas, liver and adrenals are throwing the blood sugar level back and forth from high to low. It is far preferable to eat the more slowly metabolizing complex carbohydrates such as grains, legumes, and vegetables. All of these foods have a complex structure that is more slowly broken down in the digestive process. This causes the blood sugar level to rise slowly, peak slowly and fall slowly, stabilizing the woman's moods and cravings as well as her energy.

For most women it is enough to eat these complex carbohydrates during meals, but some women may need to eat them as between-meal snacks as well in order to keep their blood sugar levels stable. Whole-grain bread spread with sesame butter is a particularly good snack for this problem.

If your craving gets out of control and you find yourself eating one sweet after another, use the macrobiotic method of stopping a sugar binge by eating mildly salty food (miso, for example), bitter food (like burdock or dandelion root), or pickled food (like umeboshi plums). These foods should stop the sugar craving immediately.

How to Beat Caffeine Addiction

If you drink three or four or more cups of coffee a day, you probably will not be able to quit abruptly because of the withdrawal headache caffeine causes. It's best to cut down by a half-cup or so a day. You can replace the coffee or tea with another warm drink, either herb tea or a roasted-grain beverage that tastes like coffee. If you drink herb teas, remember to drink a variety, because many herbs are strong substances, with untoward effects of their own if taken in excess.

Caffeine, like nicotine, is a work-drug for many people. If you have been depending on caffeine to help you work better, try meditation, repeating affirmations or exercise instead. (See the chapters on stress and exercise.)

If you depend on coffee to wake you up and help you stay alert, substitute licorice-and-ginger tea: Add two teaspoons of licorice root and two teaspoons of grated ginger root to one quart of water. Boil for five minutes and steep for fifteen minutes. This tea can be stored in the refrigerator and reheated. It should be taken in moderation (a cup or less a day).

How to Fight Chocolate Addiction

Chocolate addiction is basically sugar addiction, complicated by the fact that chocolate is a complex food, containing—in addition to sugar—fat, caffeine, mood elevators called theobromines, and the mood-stabilizing mineral magnesium. To fight a severe chocolate addiction, cut down fairly quickly, replacing the chocolate with complex carbohydrates, and supplementing the magnesium in your diet with foods high in magnesium (see page 80) and a vitamin supplement (see page 82). If you want an emotional lift, try licorice-and-ginger tea (but not more than a cup a day). Severe premenstrual chocolate binging can be controlled with the foods listed under sugar craving (mildly salty, bitter, and pickled foods).

How to Get Eating Binges Under Control

Women with weight-control problems are at higher risk of PMS. In examining the dietary habits of women with PMS, I have found that many of them binge or eat at irregular hours, particularly late at night. There are many ways to counteract the binging habit. One of the most common—and most successful—ones used by diet control centers is to offer premeasured meals to the women clients, either in the form of powdered supplements or as frozen meals. This is why so many women do well in these programs. You can set up the same type of support system in your own home by preplanning menus for each day. Decide, in effect, what you are going to eat. You can even make meals and snacks the night before. Cut up carrots and celery and package them to take to work. Pack soup in a thermos. If you crave a sweet before your period, take a piece of unsweetened carob with you, or a cookie made with fruit or apple juice instead of sugar. If a preplanned sweet is at your desk, it will eliminate the urge to run to the candy machine in midafternoon. Chew your food slowly and thoroughly. Women who binge tend to bolt down their food without chewing well. This places additional stress on the digestive tract, for it has to work hard to break down and assimilate food. Do not eat your big meal at night, for your body processes food inefficiently while you are sleeping, and you will tend to gain weight. Eat your big meal at noon and dine lightly in the evening. Keep a calendar in the kitchen and mark a star or an **X** for cheating to remind you each day of your goals. Make a tape of your own voice with your affirmations such as, "I want to eat only at mealtimes. I do not feel a need to binge. I enjoy the beauty of my lovely figure." All of these methods will help program your mind and body chemistry for success.

How to Lessen Fatigue and Improve Stamina

Many women with PMS complain of feeling spaced-out, tired and lethargic. Standard pick-me-ups like coffee, tea, or sweets only worsen the problem, but there are some foods that help build stamina and energy in the long run.

Brown-Rice Miso. Brown-rice miso is a very nutritious food that can be eaten in soup or added to other foods as a seasoning. It can be found in most good health food stores. (See page 72 for a more complete discussion.)

Burdock Root Tea. Burdock root is very strengthening for women with PMS. It is not easy to find fresh. Your best bet is to order it dried from one of the mail order sources listed on page 230. Make a tea from the dried root and drink a cup a day for the last one or two weeks of your cycle.

Dandelion Root Tea. Dandelion root tea is another strengthening tea that can be found in health food stores or ordered by mail.

Umeboshi Plum Tea. Umeboshi plum tea is a traditional Japanese tea that aids digestion and restores energy. (For the tea recipe, see page 73.)

Buckwheat. Buckwheat is a hearty grain used to provide stamina. Cereals made from buckwheat can be found in health food stores. The cooked whole grain can also be eaten in the morning. If you are particularly tired, use whole groats or buckwheat noodles as a side dish for lunch or dinner.

Biosalt. Biosalt is used by Dr. Hazel Parcell, a clinical practitioner in nutritional biochemistry, to help combat fatigue. It is a mixture of potassium and sodium that she has found to help stabilize the blood sugar level, boost adrenal function, and improve energy. It is delicious sprinkled over food. If you are particularly tired, Dr. Parcell suggests mixing a quarter teaspoon of Biosalt in six ounces of water and sipping it twice a day. Biosalt may be ordered by mail (see page 231).

Remember that eating is not the only way to increase your energy and improve your stamina. Here are some other good methods you may want to try.

Vinegar Bath. Adding apple cider vinegar to a bath can improve your superficial circulation and make you feel more alert. Add sixteen ounces of apple cider vinegar to a tub of warm water. Soak for ten minutes. Do not use soap. (Your skin may turn pink and you may notice a slight temporary plumping of your facial tissues.) Follow the bath with a few seconds under a cool shower.

Dry Brush Massage. Brushing the skin of the body below the neck in a circular motion with a dry brush is another effective way to improve superficial circulation and decrease fatigue. The massage may be followed by a lukewarm bath. Brushes for dry brush massage may be bought at many health food stores.

Deep Abdominal Breathing. Many people breathe shallowly when they are under stress and are not aware that they are decreasing their energy levels by doing so. Deep abdominal breathing is a very important means for combating fatigue, because it improves blood flow and oxygenation to the brain. (See the chapter on stress reduction for the proper method of deep abdominal breathing.)

How to Combat Periodic Weight Gain

For women who tend to accumulate weight at the time of their periods and then have a hard time taking it off, there are several vegetables that can help. (In Oriental medicine, these vegetables are thought to dissolve fatty accumulations.)

Daikon. The Oriental vegetable called daikon or daikon radish can be served grated and raw as a side dish or sliced and raw in salads. It can also be julienned or grated and steamed, and then served with tamari on the side. Many good general supermarkets now stock daikon.

Kombu. Kombu is a sea vegetable that can be used in soups, added to steamed vegetables, or served as a condiment. It can be found in Oriental groceries and health food stores.

Also, make sure that your bowels are working properly, so that you don't reabsorb fluids and waste products that should be eliminated from the body. This can cause excess weight gain. Women who have problems with constipation should be sure to include bran in their diets. One to eight tablespoons per day should suffice. Bran can be mixed with soup or water or baked into muffins.

Women who retain fluids in their tissues may be helped by mildly diuretic teas such as parsley and uva ursi.

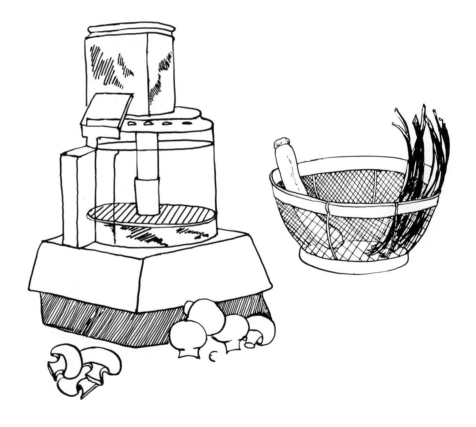

9

The Easy Way to Cook the Women's Diet

Cooking the foods on the Women's Diet is not difficult. A few small changes in your cooking utensils and methods will make it even simpler. Here is a compendium of the methods my patients and I have learned to make things easy for ourselves.

YOUR KITCHEN

The following cooking utensils are recommended for women with PMS:

Colander

The colander makes it very easy to rinse fruits and vegetables and drain foods such as pasta, tofu and salad makings. It's an inexpensive and useful kitchen item.

Food Processor

Grinding, grating, chopping, and shredding take just a few seconds with a food processor.

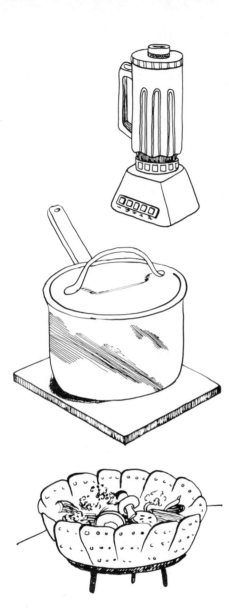

Blender

A blender is useful for puréeing vegetables and fruits, making sauces, and mixing batters for breads or cookies. It is less expensive than a food processor and can be a mainstay of your kitchen.

Stainless Steel, Enamel, or Iron Pots and Pans

Avoid aluminum pots, for the metal is toxic and can leach into your food. Avoid copper tea kettles, frying pans, etc. Copper competes with zinc, which is needed to combat acne, for binding sites in your cells. High levels of copper in the body accentuate the effect of estrogen and can cause mood changes. The PMS sufferer is more than likely to have this problem already. It does not have to be exacerbated by her cookware, which should be stainless steel, enamel, or iron.

Stainless Steel Steamer

Steaming is one of the best ways to guard the nutritional value of your vegetables and meats, since vitamins and minerals are retained in the cooking process. There are many types of steamers, but the least expensive are the stainless steel baskets. Also available are automatic electric steamers that can cook a wide range of foods, including grains.

Wok

A wok can be very useful for making one-dish meals. Grains, diced vegetables, and meat can be thrown together and

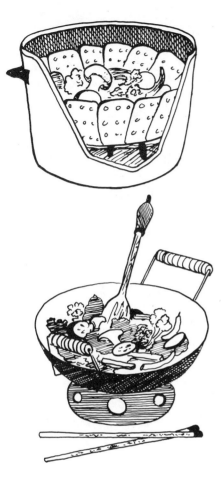

stir-fried in liquid in a few minutes. An entire meal—complete from the standpoint of nutritional content—can be made in less than ten minutes.

COOKING METHODS

Steaming

Food to be steamed is placed in a basket above boiling water. The food is cooked by steam and doesn't touch the boiling water directly. After the water has boiled a few seconds, the flame is turned low and a lid is placed on the pot to hold the steam in. Steamed food tends to have a much more interesting texture and taste than boiled food. Steaming takes no longer than preparing frozen vegetables or heating a TV dinner.

Oil-less Stir-frying

This method can replace frying in many dishes and thus eliminate a lot of fat. It can be done either in a frying pan or a wok. Instead of hot oil, use broth, bouillon, soy sauce, or water. Stir the foods into the hot liquid. This will cook them quickly and seal the juices into the food. Many vegetables contain enough natural sugar to brown naturally by this method.

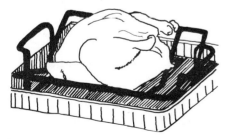

Roasting

Poultry should be roasted on a rack, spit or stand to allow the fat to run off.

Trimming and Cutting of Meat

All extra fat should be trimmed off meat. Poultry should have the skin and fat removed.

Baking

It is preferable to bake at low to moderate temperatures (325 to 375 degrees). Slow cooking preserves more nutrients and more moisture for better texture and flavor.

SHORTCUTS FOR COOKING AND STORING

You can save a lot of time by breaking up your tasks. Here are some of the methods my patients and I have worked out.

- Cook for several meals at a time. For example, prepare two soups and a stew on the weekend. They can be frozen or refrigerated in meal-size containers without losing their nutritional value.

- Many women avoid preparing dried beans because they can take hours to boil and soften. This can be discouraging if you are in a hurry. Here is a method to speed up the cooking time:

  Bring water to a boil (three cups of water for every cup of beans). Add the beans to the boiling water and cook for two minutes. Remove from the heat, partially cover the pan and let beans stand for one hour. Go about your business or chores during this time as the beans are cooking themselves. After one hour, drain and rinse with cold water and then freeze.

When you are ready to use the beans for a meal, thaw them quickly under running water. Boil five cups of water in a pot for every cup of beans. Add the beans. Lower the heat and then cook for thirty to fifty minutes. Beans will then be ready to use.

• Brown rice or grains can be prepared in large quantities. Grains store for several days in the refrigerator in a jar or plastic container. They can be reheated and used as needed for dishes. Rice is best reheated by placing it over a double boiler or in a steamer and cooking it for three to five minutes.

• Bread freezes very well and can be kept indefinitely. Slices of bread can be removed from the loaf and left to thaw gradually. They can also be placed in a toaster and warmed in a few seconds. Make sure that the bread is stored in a plastic bag and sealed so that it is airtight.

• Hot cereal can be prepared the night before. Preheat a thermos by filling it with hot water. Pour out the water. Then put three quarters of a cup of cereal and one-and-one-quarter cups of very hot water in the thermos. Put the lid on the thermos, shake it a few times, and lay it on its side. The cereal will be ready to eat by morning.

• Leafy green vegetables and other salad makings should be trimmed and washed immediately after buying. They should be stored in plastic bags and refrigerated immediately. This will not only keep them fresher, but also will leave less work for you when you cook.

• Vegetable and chicken stock can be stored in the freezer indefinitely. Freeze in small amounts so a whole pot of soup doesn't have to be defrosted for one meal and then refrozen. It can be frozen in ice cube trays.

• A combination plate such as a soup or an oil-less stir-fry
can be a complete meal in one dish and very quick to
make. An oil-less stir-fry might consist of brown rice (pre-
cooked) to which you add diced vegetables like
onions, carrots, or snow peas and meat like chicken or
shrimp; they can all be cooked together in a frying pan
with a little soy sauce, bouillon, or water. Soup can be
stored in the freezer and heated quickly. You can add
croutons, parsley, and soy bits as a garnish. A green salad
and whole grain bread can be served on the side.

10

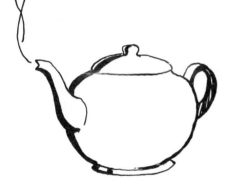

Planning and Preparing Meals

BREAKFAST

Morning seems to be the hardest part of the day for most of us. There always seems to be too much to do and not enough time. On weekdays many women skip breakfast entirely. Others eat foods like doughnuts and coffee in hopes of getting quick energy. On weekends, when most of us lounge around and rest, the hearty old American breakfast—eggs, bacon, orange juice, milk, toast, and butter—is served. Any one of these scenarios can wreak havoc for the PMS sufferer.

The Best Foods for Breakfast

Breakfast is actually the most important meal of the day. Eating a nourishing breakfast can provide the energy and sense of well-being that is so important to getting your tasks for the day done. Surprisingly enough, I've found that for most of my patients, even though breakfast is often the worst-planned meal of the day, it is also the easiest meal to restructure, because it's the meal that is most under their control. They do not have to contend with the limited choice available in a restaurant or cafeteria or the social pressure of eating with friends. Your goal should be a breakfast that is quick and easy to prepare, delicious, and useful in minimizing PMS symptoms. This is best achieved by highlighting the following foods:

Complex Carbohydrates. Complex carbohydrates are the best foods to stabilize your blood sugar and provide constant, slowly released energy throughout the day. They also help tremendously to normalize the mood swings that are so devastating to PMS sufferers. Good sources of complex carbohydrates include:

- *Hot Cereals.* As I mentioned in Chapter Five, there are many excellent grain cereals available at local health food stores. Look for cream of rye, cream of buckwheat, whole grain oatmeal, and seven- or four-grain cereals. Choose brands without added sugar. If there is no health food store near you, most supermarkets will have adequate products. Highly recommended are Wheatena, to which you can add extra bran, Maltex, and Quaker whole oatmeal (not the quick-cooking refined product). Many of the "natural cereals" from the large companies are either highly refined or highly sugared. So read the labels carefully and watch out.

- *Cold Cereals.* Again there are a large number if you patronize health food stores. These include puffed rice, corn, or millet, and unsweetened granola. At supermarkets, look for products that say "whole grain." Avoid cold cereals with added sugar.

    You can moisten your cereal with a very small amount of cow's milk or use substitutes such as goat's milk, soy milk or nut milk. Some women enjoy eating the cereals dry or with a small amount of apple juice. For sweeteners your best bet is fructose or maple syrup. They are very concentrated in flavor, so a little bit goes a long way.

- *Muffins, Breads, and Crackers.* Try muffins, breads, and crackers with applesauce, nut butter, or simple fruit preserves. Also highly recommended are the rice cakes commonly available at health food stores and now increasingly stocked at neighborhood supermarkets.

Spreads. There are many delicious spreads that are more healthful than cow's-milk butter. They often contain some vegetable oil and protein, which work in tandem with complex carbohydrates to stabilize the blood sugar level. Peanut butter (without added salt), sesame butter (which is high in calcium), and soy spreads are all good. Sesame butter is in the foreign foods department of most supermarkets and available in all health food stores. It is delicious and a wonderful source of nutrients. It is also very filling, so a little bit goes a long way. Applesauce and fruit preserves made without sugar are also good on toast, pancakes, and muffins.

Soups. Did you know that soup is a staple of the traditional breakfast in Japan? If you are used to a hearty breakfast in the morning, soup can replace traditional high-protein foods such as eggs, sausage, bacon, and steak. Soups can be either homemade or powdered, if you are short on time. Powdered soups, however, should contain neither sugar nor salt. Your best bet to combat morning fatigue is to eat legume soups such as lentil or split pea with a grain product (cereal, toast). Grains and legumes complement each other in their amino acid content and together produce a high quality protein. Also good are vegetable soup and chicken broth. For added energy I would suggest adding one teaspoon of miso to your cup of soup in the morning. Miso is a fermented soy product of Japanese origin. It is easily found in Oriental markets and health food stores. It is one of the best foods I know for increasing stamina in the morning, when many PMS sufferers are feeling low.

Beverages. Your best bet is to drink the grain-based coffee substitutes such as Pero, Postum, or Caffix, or herb teas. If anxiety and irritability are among your symptoms, teas such as chamomile and hops can take the edge off your mood.

Sample Breakfast Menus

These menus can act as guidelines for a healthful and low-stress breakfast format.

puffed rice cereal
soy milk
strawberries

buckwheat pancakes
sunflower seeds
nut milk

whole-grain waffles
blackberries
roasted grain beverage

granola (unsweetened)
nut milk
vegetable broth

bran muffin
peanut butter
apple
herb tea

oatmeal with maple syrup
pear
roasted grain beverage

whole-grain toast
sesame butter
split pea soup
herb tea

LUNCH AND DINNER

Combination Plates

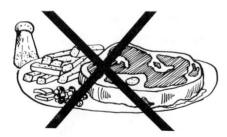

American dinners have traditionally been organized around a large piece of meat or fish. This forms the focal point, with grains and vegetables as side dishes. For the PMS sufferer it is preferable to highlight grains and vegetables and use meat more as a flavoring, cut into small pieces and

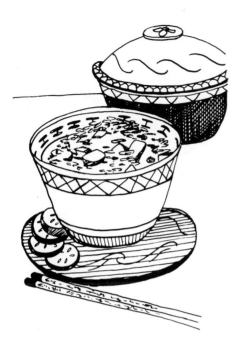

added to soups, salads, casseroles, and stir-fried dishes. Examples would include chicken soup with rice and vegetables; and tacos with beans, shredded chicken, or shrimp on a corn tortilla. With added vegetables and sauce, the taco provides three good sources of high-quality protein: meat, beans, and grain.

Casseroles

Casseroles are usually made with a cheese- or butter-based sauces, but should be made with more nutritious sauces. For example, purée vegetables such as broccoli, cauliflower, and carrots and then blend the purée with chicken broth for a creamy sauce. Arrowroot powder, rice flour, or buckwheat flakes can be added as a thickener. Tofu can also be blended into the sauce for extra creaminess.

Spices

Avoid black pepper, table salt, sugar, and monosodium glutamate (MSG). Instead use the milder herbs, such as basil, thyme, dill, and tarragon. If you must use the stronger spices, use only one half to one fourth the amount called for in the recipe.

Vegetables

Many people grew up not liking vegetables because they were poorly prepared. Cooking vegetables is an art. Here is how to prepare them so that you fall in love with them.

Leafy Green Vegetables. Kale, collard, turnip greens, mustard greens, and beet greens are packed with nutrients such as magnesium and iron that are essential to controlling premenstrual symptoms. Greens should be lightly steamed until tender but not soggy. They should never be boiled. After steaming, dress them with a mixture of olive oil, lemon juice, and a touch of sea salt. (This dressing is touted by natural healers as a liver cleanser that improves the efficiency of liver function. If this is true, the dressing can be useful for PMS sufferers. At the least, it is a delicious way to prepare greens.) Serve these vegetables as side dishes several times a week. Broccoli is also delicious when marinated in this dressing.

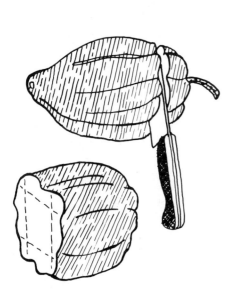

Squash. Baking squash makes it dry and stringy. There are three better ways to prepare it.

- Steam until soft, then purée the squash in a blender. The resulting purée will be soft, smooth, and a beautiful golden color. The puréeing breaks down the complex carbohydrates so that it is surprisingly sweet and delicious. This taste is similar to sweet potatoes. You may want to add nutmeg and cinnamon for extra flavor.

- Trim an acorn squash into a cube. Then cut the squash in half and remove the seeds. Steam for twenty minutes, then bake in the oven until soft. The squash will retain moisture this way and have a marvelous texture. Serve with a small amount of cinnamon or maple syrup.

- Slice the squash and sauté in olive oil, soy sauce, or broth.

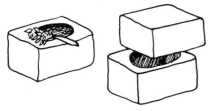

Root Vegetables. Rutabagas, turnips, parsnips and yams can be julienned (cut into long strips like french fries) and then steamed. Cook until soft but firm. Sprinkle with parsley before serving.

Root vegetables can also be steamed until soft and then puréed or whipped in a blender. Turnips cooked this way taste buttery, almost like mashed potatoes.

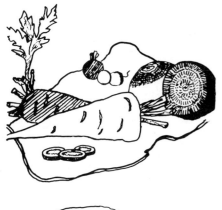

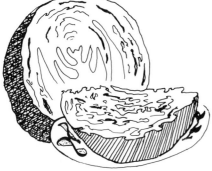

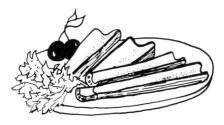

Cabbage. For an elegant but simple presentation, cut the cabbage in half, then cut wedges out of the cabbage like slices of a pie. Steam these wedges and serve each wedge on its own small side plate. Sprinkle with parsley, fennel, or caraway seeds.

Celery. Cut celery into thick french-fry-shaped sticks. Steam until soft. Serve with a garnish of pimento or tiny bits of red pepper. The red pepper may be steamed with the celery.

Salads. Ingredients should be crisp and fresh. They should be well drained in a colander or on a paper towel. Rather than cutting leaf lettuce, gently tear the leaves by hand and toss them into the salad bowl. Add the dressing just before serving or serve it on the side so that each diner can choose her own. Dark green vegetables such as romaine lettuce, endive, parsley, and red lettuce are more nutritious than iceberg lettuce. Salads can be made from a variety of raw vegetables. Don't forget turnips, beets, carrots, cauliflower, water chestnuts, snow peas, and jicama. They can be garnished with sprouts, soy bits, seeds, croutons, and nuts. Avoid store-bought salad dressings. Many contain MSG, sugar, and undesirable chemicals. Your own can be made with cold-pressed oils, lemon juice, or vinegar. Here are some good combinations:

sesame butter	sesame oil
horseradish	rice vinegar
tomato juice	green onions
mayonnaise	
	olive oil
oil	lemon juice
vinegar	garlic, basil,
avocado	and other herbs
salt	

Sample Lunch and Dinner Menus
One-Dish Meals Made with Meat

Chicken Soup
barley
chicken
carrots
celery
turnips

Turkey Stir-Fry
brown rice
turkey
broccoli
water chestnuts
tamari soy sauce

Fish Stew
fish
onions
garlic
carrots
tomato

Meals Made with Meat (three- to four-ounces)

cole slaw
sea bass
brown rice
green beans
rutabaga

romaine lettuce salad
turkey
corn bread
brussels sprouts
squash

mixed green salad
veal
whole-grain pasta
red peppers
celery

red onion and
    green pepper salad
chicken
millet
beets
broccoli

cucumber salad
sole
brown rice
mustard greens
carrots

One-Dish Meals Made without Meat

Taco
corn tortilla
pinto beans
lettuce
tomato and
   avocado garnish
onions

Lasagna
whole grain pasta
sunflower seeds
zucchini
steamed broccoli
onions
tomato sauce and cheese
   garnish (small amount)

Oil-Less Stir-Fry
brown rice
tofu
bean sprouts
green onions
soy sauce

Meals Made without Meat

Meals Organized around Soup

barley-lentil soup
rye bread
broccoli
daikon radish
applesauce

navy bean soup
kasha (buckwheat groats)
turnips
carrots
pears

mushroom soup
wild rice
green beans
stewed onions
strawberries

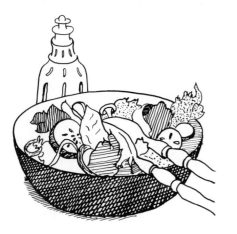

Meals Organized around Salads

mixed green salad with
sunflower-seed garnish
rye bread
soy spread

marinated vegetables (broccoli, cauliflower,
   carrots, mushrooms, and scallions) in
   vinaigrette dressing
cold pasta salad

apple and walnut salad on
   a bed of romaine lettuce
celery
bran muffins

Meals Organized around Sandwiches

tuna sandwich
on wheat bread
cole slaw

turkey sandwich
on rye bread
cole slaw

sesame butter and
   banana sandwich
   on rye bread
vegetable soup

11

The Women's Diet Cookbook

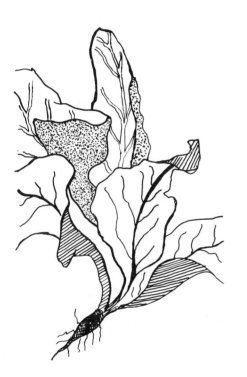

When I was first married, during my medical school and postgraduate training, I cooked by Julia Child and the *Larousse Gastronomique*. My husband and I entertained often; in one memorable year we gave thirty-five dinner parties. We and our friends all enjoyed cooking together. Many of my friendships were sealed with butter and cream, sherry and Madeira.

At the same time, in my medical studies, I was beginning to piece together the nutritional basis for many PMS symptoms. When I finally realized how badly I had been sabotaging myself, I was shocked: the wonderful lingering meals and friendly evenings were directly connected to my pain, bloating, and bad moods.

French cooking went out the window, and I started over with Oriental cooking, which uses much less fat, red meat, and milk products. Once I learned the basics of Oriental cooking, I began adapting the individual recipes by adding ingredients that corrected PMS and eliminating any that worsened it. Then I began substituting low-stress ingredients for high-stress ingredients in recipes from other cuisines, especially recipes for desserts, which for me were among the hardest things to give up.

Eventually, without my really planning it, a cuisine evolved that used only foods that were good for women. I began sharing my recipes with my patients, and their enthusiastic responses (and requests for a cookbook) got me started on this book.

When it was time to test the recipes for the book, I did all the cooking myself and enjoyed it very much. Having a house full of happy tasters reminded me of the good old days—except that this time the food was good for us and easy to prepare. It was very gratifying to see older men and little babies all enjoying the food made for women with PMS. (One of the most enthusiastic tasters was my ten-month-old little girl, who couldn't get enough of the nut milk.) So I don't think you have to worry about sharing your diet with your family and friends.

SOUPS

Chicken Soup   *Serves 8*

> ½ chicken breast
> 1 to 1½ quarts chicken stock
> 1 onion
> 2 large carrots
> ¼ to 1 teaspoon basil
> sea salt to taste

Chop vegetables into bite-sized pieces. Place them in pot. Add chicken breast, chicken stock, and water. Bring to a boil with pot uncovered. Turn heat to low, cover pot, and let soup cook until vegetables are soft. Add basil and sea salt to taste.

Variation: Add any or a combination of the ingredients listed below. All have high nutritional value for women with PMS and will add to the flavor of the soup.

⅛ head of cabbage, diced
¼ cup green beans, chopped into small pieces
¼ cup green peas
½ cup turnips, chopped
4 leaves kale
5 sprigs parsley
½ cup red beans
4 ounces corn elbow pasta
4 ounces whole wheat elbow pasta

Miso Soup *Serves 4*

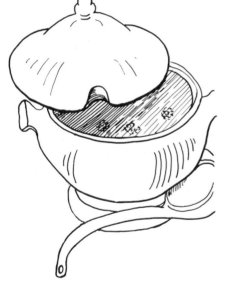

4½ cups water
2 carrots, sliced
1 onion, sliced
¼ head cabbage, chopped
4 tablespoons red miso
2 tablespoons scallions or parsley, minced

Heat ½ cup water in pot. Add onion and carrots and cook for 7 minutes. Add another ½ cup of water and the cabbage and cook for 5 more minutes. Add the remainder of the water, cover pot, and bring to a boil. Turn heat to low and simmer for 15 minutes. Cream the miso with a little cooking water, then add to the pot and remove from heat. Sprinkle with scallions or parsley to serve.

Lentil Soup

Serves 4

1 cup lentils
½ onion, chopped
½ cup carrots, chopped
1 to 1½ quarts water
2 to 3 tablespoons brown rice miso or
 ¼–½ teaspoon sea salt

Wash lentils. Put lentils, onions, carrots, water, and miso in a pot. Bring to a boil, then turn heat to low, cover pot, and simmer for 45 minutes, or until lentils are soft.

Split Pea Soup

Serves 4

1 cup split peas
½ onion, chopped
1 small carrot, sliced
1 quart water
¼ to ½ teaspoon sea salt

Wash peas. Place peas, onion, and carrot in a pot. Add the water. Bring to a boil, then turn heat to low and cover pot. Cook for 45 minutes. Add sea salt and continue to cook until peas are soft. Soup may be cooled and then puréed in a blender if you prefer a creamy texture.

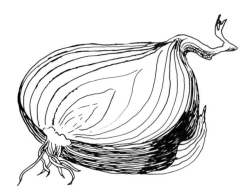

Summer Squash Soup

Serves 6

4 yellow summer squash
1 quart water
1 onion, chopped
¼ to ½ teaspoon sea salt
  (miso or tamari may be substituted)

Place chopped squash and onion in a pot. Add the water, bring to a boil and then turn heat to low and cover pot. Cook for 15 minutes over low flame. Add sea salt and continue cooking for another 15 minutes, until vegetables are soft. Let cool and then purée in blender. Garnish with sliced scallions or minced parsley.

Artichoke Broth

Serves 4

1 chopped onion
4 artichokes
1½ quarts water
½ teaspoon sea salt
Vegit or Vegesal (seasoning mixtures
  available from health food stores) to taste

Place the ingredients in a pot and cover with water. Bring to a boil and then turn heat to low. Simmer for 1½ hours. Do not overcook. (If cooked too long, broth may become bitter.)

Vegetable Soup *Serves 4 to 6*

1 onion, chopped
1 stalk celery, chopped
1 turnip, chopped
½ leek, chopped
2 carrots, chopped
¼ bunch parsley, chopped
5 mushrooms, sliced
½ tablespoon fennel
1 bay leaf
½ tablespoon thyme
¼–½ teaspoon sea salt
1½ quarts artichoke broth

Place all ingredients in a pot. Cover with the artichoke broth from the previous recipe. Bring to a boil, then turn heat to low. Cook for 2 hours. Strain out half the vegetables and herbs. Pour the remainder of the soup and vegetables into individual serving dishes. Garnish with finely chopped vegetables.

SALADS

Watercress Salad *Serves 4*

2 bunches watercress
6 ounces fresh bean sprouts
2 teaspoons scallion, finely chopped
½ tablespoon sunflower seeds
vinaigrette dressing

Wash watercress. Remove the large stems and place the rest in a bowl. Add bean sprouts and scallion. Toss the salad. Add the sunflower seeds and vinaigrette dressing and toss again. Serve immediately.

Tofu-Wild Rice Salad

Serves 4

6 ounces tofu
2 cups cooked wild rice
3 scallions, chopped
¼ to ½ cup minced parsley
½ green pepper, minced
herbal oil and vinegar dressing

Cut tofu into bite-size pieces. Combine with all the other ingredients in a bowl. Mix with your favorite herbal oil-and-vinegar dressing to taste. Note: Brown rice may be substituted for wild rice.

Brown Rice and Chicken Salad

Serves 4

2 cups cooked brown rice
½ boiled or roasted chicken breast, diced
1 green onion, diced
¼ cup raisins
1½ ounces blanched almonds
¼ cup peas, cooked
¼ cup green pepper
¼ cup celery

Combine all ingredients in a bowl. The salad may be dressed with a vinaigrette dressing or with a dressing made by combining 1½ tablespoons seasoned rice wine vinegar, ½ teaspoon Worcestershire sauce and 2½ tablespoons mayonnaise.

Lentil Salad

1 cup lentils
2 cups water
½ teaspoon sea salt
¼ cup celery, finely chopped
¼ cup red onion, finely chopped
¼ cup black olives, finely chopped
2 to 3 tablespoons wine vinegar
3 tablespoons olive oil
1 teaspoon basil

Wash lentils and combine with water in a pot. Cook for ½ hour or until lentils are soft.

Combine all ingredients in a bowl. Toss with wine vinegar, olive oil, and basil.

Romaine Salad

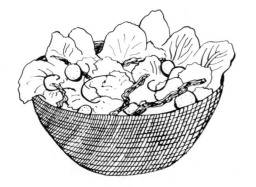

1 head romaine lettuce
⅛ head red cabbage, chopped
4 radishes, sliced
1 small carrot, grated
oil and vinegar to taste

Combine all ingredients in a bowl and toss with oil and vinegar.

Miso Salad Dressing

Makes 1½ cups

> 1 cup warm water
> 1 teaspoon miso
> ½ minced garlic clove
> juice of ¼ to ½ lemon
> dash cayenne pepper
> ½ cup tahini (sesame butter)

Dissolve miso in warm water. Place in blender with remaining ingredients. Blend until smooth. Yield: approximately 1½ cups. (For thinner consistency, add more water. For dip consistency, use less water.)

Variation: 1 to 3 teaspoons seasoned rice wine vinegar may be added for sweetness.

VEGETABLES AND GRAINS

Note: You may want to vary steaming times depending on whether you like a firm or a soft texture.

Celery Julienne

Serves 4

> 6 stalks celery
> 2 tablespoons sweet red pepper, chopped

Cut the celery into small strips (like french-fried potatoes). Steam for 15 to 20 minutes, or until tender. Drain and toss with red pepper.

Steamed Leeks
Serves 4

8 medium leeks
2 tablespoons red onion, minced

Remove and discard green tops of leeks and rinse thoroughly. Cut each root end into two pieces. Steam for 15 to 20 minutes or until tender. Sprinkle onion on top before serving.

Diced Carrots with Peas
Serves 4

1½ cups chicken stock
1 cup green peas
1 cup carrots, diced

Heat the chicken broth to boiling, then turn heat to low. Add the peas and carrots and simmer for 30 minutes or until vegetables are tender.

Cauliflower with Parsley
Serves 4

1 head medium cauliflower
3 to 4 tablespoons fresh parsley, finely chopped

Break the cauliflower into small flowerets. Steam for 10 minutes or until tender. Toss with fresh parsley.

Broccoli with Lemon
Serves 4

1 pound broccoli
juice of ½ lemon

Cut the broccoli into small flowerets; steam for 15 minutes or until tender. Squeeze lemon juice over broccoli.

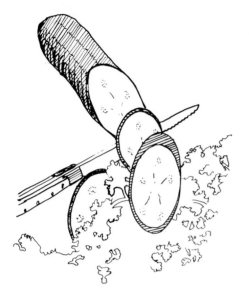

Zucchini with Scallions

Serves 4

2 medium zucchini
2 teaspoons scallions, chopped
1 teaspoon parsley, finely chopped

Dice the zucchini. Place in an ungreased shallow pan and sprinkle with the other ingredients. Cover pan and bake at 350 degrees for 30 minutes.

Savory Bean Sprouts

Serves 4

1 cup chicken stock
1½ cups bean sprouts
1 cup mushrooms, sliced

Heat the chicken stock over a low flame for 5 minutes. Add the bean sprouts and mushrooms. Simmer for 10 minutes.

Whipped Acorn Squash

Serves 4

2 acorn squash
2 to 3 ounces apple juice
pinch ground cinnamon

Peel and cut acorn squash into large pieces. Steam until tender. Place in blender, add apple juice and cinnamon, and purée. You may also want to add water in small amounts until smooth and creamy.

Summer Squash and Peas

Serves 4

2 to 3 small summer squash, diced
1 cup peas

Steam peas for 10 minutes. Add squash and steam vegetables together for 15 minutes or until tender. Drain and serve.

Vegetable Purée #1

Serves 4

3 to 4 carrots, chopped
⅛ head cabbage, chopped
1 cup peas

Steam carrots for 15 minutes, add rest of vegetables and steam another 15 minutes, until soft. Place in blender and purée. Slowly add water until smooth and creamy.

Vegetable Purée #2

Serves 4

4 summer squash, chopped
1 medium beet, chopped

Steam beet for 15 minutes. Add squash to the pot and steam the vegetables together for 15 more minutes, or until soft. Purée in blender.

Brown Rice

Serves 4

1 cup brown rice
2 cups cold water
½ teaspoon sea salt

Wash rice with cold water. Combine all ingredients in a cooking pot. Bring ingredients to a rapid boil. Turn flame to low, cover, and cook without stirring about 25 to 35 minutes, until rice is soft. Resist the temptation to check before 20 minutes, since that lets out too much steam.

Kasha   *Serves 4*

> 1 cup kasha (buckwheat groats)
> 3¼ cups water
> pinch salt

Bring ingredients to a boil, lower heat, and simmer for 25 minutes or until soft. The grains should be fluffy like rice. Note: Kasha is especially good for women with PMS. For breakfast, blend in blender with water till it is a "cream." Add almond milk, sesame milk, or sunflower milk; and cinnamon, apple butter, ginger, raisins, or berries.

MEATS AND FISH

Glazed Chicken   *Serves 4*

> 4 chicken breasts, approximately 3 ounces each
> 2 cups chicken stock
> 2 tablespoons dry white wine
> pinch thyme
> ½ cup carrots, finely julienned
> ½ cup celery, diced
> ½ cup mushrooms, sliced

Remove skin and fat from chicken. Place in pan and brown in 500-degree oven for 5 minutes. Combine the chicken stock and wine. Simmer the mixture in a separate pot for 10 minutes. Pour the chicken stock and wine over the chicken. Add the thyme and carrots. Cover and cook for 20 minutes or until carrots are tender. Remove the chicken pieces. Add mushrooms and celery to the sauce; simmer and reduce by half. Cover each chicken piece with the sauce and serve hot.

Chicken with Lemon and Ginger

Serves 4

4 chicken breasts, approximately 3 ounces each
1 cup chicken stock
1 tablespoon soy sauce
1 tablespoon lemon juice
¼ teaspoon garlic powder
freshly grated ginger

Remove skin and fat from chicken. Combine chicken stock, soy sauce, lemon juice, and garlic in a skillet. Add grated ginger to taste. Simmer the broth until it is reduced by half. Marinate the chicken in this mixture for 45 minutes. Place chicken and marinade in a pan and bake at 350 degrees for 40 minutes.

Cold Salmon Plate

Serves 4

4 fillets of salmon, 3 ounces each
1 cup water
2 tablespoons lemon juice
1 tablespoon dry white wine
4 cups shredded lettuce
8 lemon wedges
fresh parsley sprigs
1 small red onion, separated into rings

Combine water, lemon juice, and wine in skillet and heat. Place the salmon in the hot liquid. Cover and poach for 10 minutes or until salmon flakes easily with a fork. Remove the fish and let it chill in the refrigerator. Arrange the lettuce, lemon wedges, and parsley sprigs on individual plates. Place the chilled salmon in the center of each plate, top with the onion rings, and serve.

Poached Salmon   *Serves 4*

    4 fillets of salmon, 3 ounces each
    1 cup water
    1 lemon
    1 tablespoon onion, diced
    1 tablespoon carrot, diced
    2 ounces V8 juice

Combine the water and the juice of one lemon in skillet and heat. Place the salmon in the hot liquid and sprinkle with diced vegetables. Cover and poach for 6 to 8 minutes or until salmon flakes easily with a fork. Remove the fish and keep it warm. Add the V8 juice to the stock and reduce the liquid by one half. Cover the salmon with the sauce and serve hot.

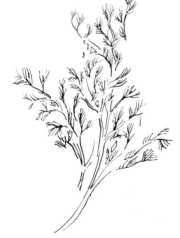

Broiled Trout with Dill   *Serves 4*

    2 fresh trout, about 8 ounces each
    2 tablespoons lemon juice
    chopped fresh dill (dried if fresh is unavailable)

Slice each trout in half and bone. This will make four fillets. Sprinkle the fillets with lemon juice and dill. Place the trout in a broiler pan. Broil for 5 or 6 minutes or until done.

Marinated Fish

Serves 4

12 ounces rock cod or other firm white fish
2½ tablespoons olive oil
2 lemons
10 bay leaves, broken in half

Cut fish into 1-inch cubes. Sprinkle 1½ teaspoons of olive oil and the juice of one lemon over the fish. Add the bay leaves, toss, and let mixture marinate for 15 minutes. Heat the remaining tablespoon of oil over medium-high heat. Cut the remaining lemon, including rind, into ¾-inch pieces. Add lemon pieces to oil, turn heat to low, and cover pot. Sauté lemon wedges until golden brown. Remove and cool. Thread 4 skewers with fish, lemon pieces, and bay leaves. Or place fish, lemon pieces, and bay leaves in a broiling pan. Broil for 10 minutes. If using skewers, turn to brown all sides.

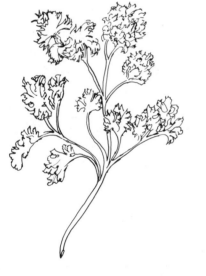

Poached Flounder

Serves 4

4 flounder fillets, 3 ounces each
2 cups water
2 shallots, chopped
2 sprigs parsley
1 small stalk celery, chopped
1 bay leaf
1 clove

Combine water, shallots, parsley, celery, bay leaf, and clove in a pot. Cover and simmer for 10 minutes. Strain. Gently add the flounder to the liquid. Cover the pot and simmer for 10 minutes or until fish is tender.

Halibut in Cashew Milk
Serves 4

4 halibut steaks, 3 ounces each
¾ cup fish stock or water
2 tablespoons dry white wine
1 shallot, minced
½ teaspoon arrowroot powder
⅓ cup cashew milk (see page 135)
1 teaspoon lemon juice

Combine the fish stock, wine, and shallot in a pot. Heat to boiling. Cover pot and then simmer 5 to 10 minutes. Place the halibut in the liquid and poach for 10 minutes. Lift the fish out carefully with a slotted spoon and keep it warm. Combine the arrowroot powder with the cashew milk. Mix it slowly into the hot fish stock, stirring constantly until the sauce is the consistency of a thin gravy. Season with lemon juice. Return the halibut to the sauce and simmer for 2 minutes.

ONE-DISH MEALS

Almond Chicken
Serves 4

3 cups brown rice, cooked
1 cup raw, boned chicken breasts, cubed
¼ cup blanched almonds
¾ cup celery, finely chopped
½ cup water
tamari soy sauce
1 teaspoon sesame or safflower oil

Sauté celery in water and oil over a low flame for 20 minutes or until tender. Add chicken and almonds. Continue cooking for 5 minutes or until chicken is done. Transfer to a serving dish and toss with rice and tamari soy sauce to taste.

Shrimp with Snow Peas

Serves 4

3 cups brown rice, cooked
¾ cup shrimp, cooked and shelled
1 cup snow peas, steamed
¼ cup water
tamari soy sauce
1 teaspoon sesame or safflower oil

Combine shrimp and snow peas in a large frying pan
with water and oil. Cook over low flame for 5 minutes. (Add
extra water to pan if needed.) Add rice to pan and mix.
Heat for 5 minutes or until warm. Transfer to serving dish and
toss with tamari soy sauce to taste.

Tacos

Serves 4

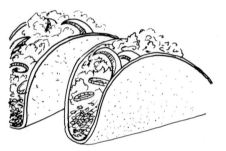

4 corn tortillas
1 pound pinto beans, cooked and puréed
½ avocado, thinly sliced
¼ yellow onion, finely chopped
6 tablespoons salsa
½ head red or romaine lettuce, chopped

Warm tortillas and beans in separate pans. Place tortillas
on individual serving dishes and spread with beans. Garnish
with avocado and onion, then cover each taco with lettuce
and 1½ tablespoons of salsa.

SPREADS

Tofu-and-Peanut-Butter Spread *Makes 1½ cups*

> ½ cup tofu, drained
> 1 cup peanut butter
> 1 to 2 tablespoons honey

Blend all ingredients in a blender or food processor.

Apple-Spice Butter *Makes 2 cups*

> 1 pound apples, peeled, quartered, and cored
> ¼ to ½ cup water
> ½ teaspoon cinnamon
> ⅛ teaspoon cloves
> ¼ teaspoon ginger
> 1 to 2 tablespoons honey

Cook apples in butter until soft. Add water and cook for 5 to 10 minutes. Add spices and honey to pan. Stir to mix. Cool. Blend in blender or food processor until smooth.

DESSERTS

Desserts are treats and can make life more fun, but commercially made goods that contain sugar, milk, butter, white flour, and other high-stress ingredients are not for the woman who wants to avoid PMS. Fortunately, there are ways to have dessert without triggering your symptoms:

- Substitute low-stress ingredients for high-stress ingredients in your regular recipes. This means replacing sugar, white flour, and dairy products with equivalent foods.

- Use special recipes that are already modified for PMS.

Substitutes for Sugar

- *Cut the amount of sweetener in your recipes by one-half to one-third.* Most recipes use too much sugar. Our taste buds have become addicted to it over the years, but as you reduce your addiction you will learn to enjoy more subtle flavors.

- *Substitute more concentrated sweeteners.* These have a sweeter taste per quantity used than table sugar. This will allow you to cut down on the actual amount of sugar used in a recipe.

$\frac{3}{4}$ cup sugar = $\frac{1}{2}$ cup honey
= $\frac{1}{4}$ cup molasses
= $\frac{1}{2}$ cup maple syrup
= $\frac{1}{2}$ ounce barley malt

If you use a concentrated sweetener in place of sugar in an ordinary recipe, reduce the liquid content in the recipe by $\frac{1}{4}$ cup. If no liquid is used in the recipe, add 3 to 4 tablespoons of flour for each $\frac{3}{4}$ cup of concentrated sweetener.

- *Substitute fruit for sugar in pastries.* In making muffins and cookies, you may want to try deleting sugar altogether and adding extra fruit and nuts. Besides being good for you, these are good treats for children who want to take cookies with them for school lunch. You will find several recipes for cookies without sugar in the following section.

$\frac{3}{4}$ cup sugar = 1 cup apple butter
= 2 cups apple juice

Substitutes for Dairy Products

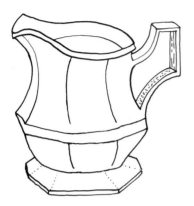

Substitutes can be used in recipes that call for the use of cow's milk. Health food stores and some chain stores carry soy milk, often in both powdered and liquid form. Add liquid acidophilus culture (used in yogurt-making) to soy milk, as it is difficult for some people to digest. Acidophilus is available in health food stores. Nut milks are occasionally available in powdered form. The following substitutes for milk can be made easily at home, and are so good they are addictive.

Nut Milk
Makes 1¼ cups

½ cup blanched almonds or cashews
1 tablespoon honey or rice syrup
1 cup warm water

Combine nuts, honey, and 1 cup of warm water in blender. Slowly add remaining water and blend until creamy. If you like a thinner milk, add 1 to 3 ounces more warm water.

Oat Milk
Makes 1¾ to 2 cups

¼ cup rolled oats
2 cups water
⅓ banana
¼ teaspoon cinnamon
2 ounces apple juice
pinch of sea salt

Combine oats and hot water in a pot. Simmer in covered pot for 20 minutes. Whip in blender with remaining ingredients until smooth and creamy.

Sesame Milk

Makes 1⅓ cups

½ cup apple juice
½ cup water
3 ice cubes
3 tablespoons tahini (sesame butter)
½ banana

Combine all ingredients in blender. This makes a delicious beverage.

Tofu Whipped Cream

Makes 2½ cups

2 cups tofu
2 cups warm water, with a pinch of sea salt
¼ cup honey
3 tablespoons tahini (sesame butter) or almond butter
1 teaspoon vanilla
¼ to ½ cup apple juice

Drop tofu into warm salted water. Remove from heat immediately. Place tofu in blender and combine with remaining ingredients. (Add apple juice slowly as cream is blending until mixture is smooth.)

Substitutes for Other Common High-Stress Ingredients

1 cup white flour = 1 cup whole wheat flour minus
2 tablespoons
½ teaspoon salt = 1 tablespoon miso
1 square chocolate = ¾ tablespoon powdered carob
1½ cups cocoa = 1 cup powdered carob

I've used these substitutions in many favorite recipes that were full of rich ingredients. The substitutions are very easy to make, so instead of throwing out your favorite recipes, try it yourself and continue to enjoy your old favorites in a more nutritious form.

Oatmeal Cookies *Makes about 3 dozen*

¼ cup honey
½ cup margarine
1 egg, slightly beaten
2 teaspoons vanilla
½ teaspoon salt
½ cup whole wheat flour
¾ teaspoon baking powder
1 cup wheat germ
1½ cup rolled oats
¾ cup raisins
¾ cup chopped nuts or toasted sunflower seeds

Preheat oven to 375 degrees. Mix margarine and honey until creamy. Combine with egg, vanilla, and salt and blend.

Mix flour, baking powder, wheat germ, and rolled oats with a fork. Add the remaining ingredients. A few teaspoons of water may be added until dough is of proper consistency.

Spoon onto greased cookie sheets and flatten each cookie slightly with a spoon. Bake for 10 to 12 minutes.

Tea Cookies *Makes 3½ dozen*

   2½ cups whole wheat flour
   ¼ teaspoon sea salt
   1½ teaspoons baking powder
   ½ cup margarine
   ¼ cup water
   ½ teaspoon vanilla
   ¼ cup honey

Preheat oven to 325 degrees.

Sift the dry ingredients together. Cream the margarine and combine it with ⅛ cup water, vanilla, and honey. Combine the wet and dry ingredients.

Knead the dough into a ball, adding the rest of the water as needed to achieve a firm texture.

Chill the dough for 1 hour and roll it to ¾-inch thick. Cut to desired shapes with a knife or cookie cutters. Transfer to greased cookie sheets and bake for 5 minutes.

Variations: Cookies may be varied by substituting orange juice for water or by adding ½ cup crushed almonds, walnuts, raisins, or poppy seeds.

Pie Crust Dough *Makes 1 crust (double to make 2)*

   1 cup whole wheat flour
   ½ cup whole wheat pastry flour
   ½ cup wheat germ
   1 teaspoon sea salt
   ½ teaspoon cinnamon
   4 ounces margarine, at room temperature
   4 tablespoons water

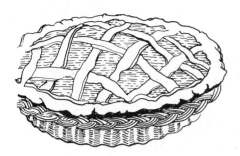

Preheat oven to 400 degrees.

Combine dry ingredients in a bowl. Mix the margarine into the dry ingredients, using either your fingers or a fork to break it into little pieces.

Form the dough into a ball with your hands, adding water as needed. Refrigerate for 20 minutes.

Roll the pie dough to the size of your pie pan, and then line the pie pan.

Apple Pie
Serves 8

> double Pie Crust Dough recipe
> 4 to 5 apples, chopped
> 2 teaspoons cinnamon
> pinch sea salt
> 2 tablespoons arrowroot powder
> ½ cup apple juice
> 1 egg yolk

Make the Pie Crust Dough and divide into two equal pieces. Roll out one piece for bottom crust and place in an oiled pie pan. Cover other piece with a damp towel.

Combine chopped fruit, cinnamon, and sea salt. Set aside.

Dissolve arrowroot powder in apple juice. Stir until they are well combined. (You may want to heat the mixture.)

Pour arrowroot mixture over fruit and blend well. Let sit for a few minutes.

Place filling in pie pan.

Roll out top crust. Cover fruit mixture with crust. Prick crust with fork and glaze with egg yolk.

Bake at 350 degrees for 30 minutes or until fruit is soft.

Blackberry Cream Pie

Serves 8

single recipe Pie Crust Dough (from page 138)
2 cups blackberries (or strawberries, raspberries,
   blueberries, or boysenberries)
1½ cups Tofu Whipped Cream (from page 136)

Make a single recipe of Pie Crust Dough. Line a pie pan with the dough and bake for 10 to 12 minutes.
Place berries in pie pan and cover with Tofu Whipped Cream.

Cashew Ice Milk

Serves 6 to 8

½ cup water
agar-agar flakes (poured to the 3-ounce mark
   in a measuring cup)
2 cups apple juice
2 egg yolks
1 cup cashew milk
2 tablespoons honey
½ teaspoon vanilla

Agar-agar is a gelatin made from seaweed. It is used as a thickening agent and can be found in most health food stores.
Combine agar-agar with water and cook over a low flame until it dissolves.
Combine agar-agar, apple juice, cashew milk, vanilla, and honey.
Combine egg yolks with a few teaspoons of the mixture. Add this to the rest of the mixture. Cook at low heat until thickened, stirring continuously.
Pour mixture into individual serving bowls and freeze.

Pound Cake

Serves 8

2½ cups whole wheat pastry flour
½ teaspoon baking soda
1½ teaspoons baking powder
½ teaspoon sea salt
1 teaspoon vanilla
⅓ cup honey
½ cup margarine
2 eggs
1 cup nut or sesame milk

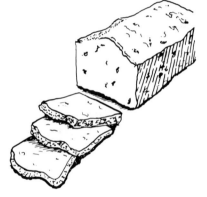

Preheat oven to 350 degrees. Sift together flour, baking soda, baking powder and salt.

Cream margarine, honey, and vanilla together.

Separate eggs. Beat the yolks and add to honey and margarine. Slowly add sifted ingredients to egg mixture with the nut or soy milk.

Beat egg whites until stiff peaks form and fold them into the dough. Place dough in well-greased pan and bake for 30 to 40 minutes or until a knife inserted in center of cake is clean when removed.

Applesauce Loaf

Serves 8

1½ cups whole wheat flour
½ cup wheat germ
½ teaspoon salt
½ teaspoon baking powder
½ teaspoon baking soda
¼ cup honey
½ cup unsweetened applesauce
½ cup margarine

Preheat oven to 375 degrees. Combine dry ingredients in a bowl.

Cream margarine and honey together. Add applesauce, mixing well.

Combine all ingredients. Place in a well-greased loaf pan. Bake for 30 to 45 minutes. Test with knife to see if loaf is done.

Adapting the Women's Diet for Pregnancy or Menopause

The Women's Diet is excellent for pregnancy and menopause if it is adapted slightly (as, in fact, any diet should be) to take into account the special dietary needs of those periods in our lives. Calcium is especially important: for pregnant women and nursing mothers because the developing baby puts additional demands on the mother's own supply; and for women in menopause because the decrease in hormone levels tends to cause demineralization of the bones. The pregnant woman also needs large amounts of iron in her diet because her blood volume is expanding tremendously, creating a tendency toward anemia.

For both pregnant women and women in menopause, sea vegetables such as dulse and kelp are important because their rich supply of iodine and trace minerals provides nutrients essential for normal endocrine function (especially of the thyroid).

For more specific information, consult books on these topics.

12

How to Reduce the Stress in Your Life

Women with PMS seem to be especially susceptible to environmental stress during the premenstrual period. Little irritations that normally wouldn't bother them assume monumental importance. They become anxious, irritable, or angry at the world around them. Unfortunately, this emotional sensitivity is very common, affecting more than 80 percent of women with PMS.

I remember as a teenager hearing for the first time the saying, "She's on the rag." This meant that a woman was having her period. It also meant that she was being irritable and difficult. The saying reflects the underlying cultural belief that women are innately unstable and mercurial, victims of their fluctuating chemistry.

This was the attitude of most of the gynecological textbooks that I read when I was a medical student. Most books suggested that women had a natural tendency toward hysteria. In addition, women who noted mood swings premenstrually were said to be poorly adapted and resentful of their feminine role or to be punishing themselves for their budding sexuality. There was no curiosity about whether there might be a physiological reason for these symptoms. All women, in effect, were lumped together with the same diagnosis. There was no awareness of the role that nutrition and other environmental factors play in determining people's body chemistry.

Since all the affected women were considered to be neurotic, the standard treatment was psychotherapy and tranquilizers. Many patients listened to their doctors' diagnoses and spent years popping tranquilizers or on a psychiatrist's couch. With psychotherapy, many women reported greater insight about their unconscious processes, but their sensitivity to stress remained. This left them with a feeling of helplessness: they had tried all of the usual medical therapies and they hadn't worked. Little effort was made to teach women how to manage stress on a practical basis.

We know now that the emotional stress symptoms of PMS are the result of a *combination* of factors. They are a response to many physical, environmental, and mental stresses. We also see that the fact that they are common does not mean that they are normal. What it does mean is that a lot of women have poor living habits. As we have seen, the symptoms of PMS can be greatly corrected with proper nutrition. With a physician's help, they can also be corrected by medications such as progesterone and the antiprostaglandin drugs. But it is also very important to learn to manage social stress.

If your metabolism is already burdened chemically and renders you hypersensitive to cyclical changes in your hormones, it is important not to add to the problem by setting up a stressful personal environment. The questions in the test on page 52 are an indication of how much stress there is in your environment. Most of the women I see in my medical practice feel that they could do better. They feel that they could find ways to improve the quality of their environment. Even women who are completely happy with their professional and personal lives feel that they could learn to manage stress better. They have become tired of feeling extremely angry, anxious, or irritable during their premenstrual period.

Many of my patients have asked me about techniques for coping better with stress. Over the last nine years, I have worked out a strategy that seems to work. I send some women for counseling or psychotherapy, but the majority are looking for practical ways to manage stress on their own. They want to take responsibility for learning to handle their own problems—looking at their methods of dealing with stress, learning techniques to improve their habits and then practicing these techniques on a regular basis. I find this self-help way to be the most effective of all.

THE PHYSIOLOGY OF STRESS

Your reaction to stress is partly determined by the sensitivity of your autonomic nervous system. The nervous system consists of the brain, the spinal cord, and the peripheral nerves. It is divided by function into two parts: the voluntary nervous system and the involuntary (or autonomic) nervous system.

The voluntary nervous system manages activity in the conscious domain. For example, if you place your hand on a hot stove, pain fibers will trigger a response that is sent to the brain. The brain sends back an immediate response telling you to move your hand before you burn yourself. You then pull your hand away, fast.

The autonomic nervous system regulates functions that the average person is usually unaware of, such as the circulation of the blood, muscle tension, pulse rate, respiration, and glandular function. The autonomic nervous system is divided into two parts that oppose and complement each other. They are called the sympathetic and parasympathetic nervous systems, and they control the upper and lower limits of your physiology. For example, if excitement speeds up the heart rate too much, it is the parasympathetic nervous system's job to act as a control circuit and slow it down. If the heart slows down too much, then it is the sympathetic nervous system's job to speed it up.

Many women with PMS have overreactive sympathetic nervous systems that are much worse during the second half of their cycle. An easily triggered sympathetic nervous system is fine if you are driving your car on the expressway on Saturday night and need to be on the lookout for drunken drivers. Your muscles tense and your blood vessels constrict so you can react to an emergency. The problem with many women who have PMS is that their sympathetic nervous systems are *always* in a state of readiness to react to a crisis. This puts them in a constant state of tension or "fight or flight." They tend to react to small stresses the same way they react to real emergencies. Their adrenal glands increase their output of adrenalin and cortisone, adjusting the body chemistry to meet the crisis. Their hearts speed up, their pulses race, and their neck and shoulder muscles tense. The energy that accumulates in the body to meet this "emergency" must then be discharged, and it is. They yell at the children or they kick the dog and their systems come into balance once again.

Macro-Stress. Two types of stress have a significant impact on people's health: major life changes and small everyday irritants. Major life changes include such important events as marriage, divorce, birth of a child, and loss of a job. Other events may be totally outside of your control but can affect you just as strongly. These include the death of a parent or an automobile accident for which you are not at fault. Human beings can adapt to change only up to a certain point without its taking a toll on their health. Even happy situations like the birth of a child mean making accommodations in your life. They take energy and require a period of adjustment.

When more than one important stress occurs in a short period of time, the effects are cumulative. This idea was developed by Dr. Thomas Holmes and his co-workers at the University of Washington Medical School. Holmes developed the Life Change Index based on a system of points: the more serious the stress, the more points were assigned to it. Thus the death of a spouse was given 100 points and considered to be much more traumatic than a change in a person's work hours, which was given only 20 points. Major life changes during a two-year period were totaled. A score of 300 points or more indicated a serious major life stress. A person with such a high score was shown to be at extremely high risk for major illness. A person with a score between 200 and 299 was thought to be at medium risk and a person scoring under 200 points at low risk.

Few of my patients date the onset of their PMS to major life changes, but all agree that major life changes, when they occurred, worsened their symptoms.

If you have not already answered the questions in the Major Stress Evaluation (based on the Holmes Life Change Index) on page 52, it would be a good idea to do that now.

Micro-Stress. While the Life Change Index is very useful in evaluating the seriousness of major changes, it is unable to assess each person's individual reaction pattern. For example, the loss of a job can be a very serious handicap and is undoubtedly a stress for everyone. However, one person might respond to it with illness and depression, while another would take it as a challenge for personal growth. Perhaps more significant in determining your resiliency in dealing with stress is how you manage little everyday irritations or micro-stresses. These can include a flat tire, missing a bus, being late for an appointment, a child's crying, overcooking a casserole, and a multitude of other happenings. We each have our own list of "hot spots" that seem to exasperate us out of proportion to the incident itself. The micro-stresses in themselves may be insignificant, but these small incidents add up. On a daily basis they can be responsible for more wear and tear than the large and dramatic life changes that Dr. Holmes describes.

It will help you to become aware of how you deal with these irritations. Does tension build up in your body? Does your breath become shallow as you become more upset, or do you begin deep breathing and exercising at the first signs of stress? Do you meditate to calm your mind? Many of my patients do not recognize their own early signs of stress. They are not aware that they are upset until the feelings become very strong. Then they smoke, eat too much, take pills, or become cranky and irritable. For most of us, effective stress management is something that has to be learned.

It is important that you evaluate your areas of micro-stress. If you have not already taken the test on page 54, turn back and do it now. If you have already taken it, it would be a good idea to go back over it for a moment.

What Stress Does to Your Body

Now that you have evaluated the areas in your life that produce stress, it is important to see how stress localizes in your body. In most people it causes tension in the muscles which is perceived as a tightness, soreness, or aching. The chronic tension obstructs the blood flow to that area of the body, cutting off the flow of oxygen to the tissues. The cells do not receive the nutrients that they need to function properly. As a result, the muscles function at a low energy level. Toxic wastes cannot be disposed of efficiently and lactic acid accumulates. This leads to fatigue. These aches and pains are your body's signal to you that you need to relax. The test on page 51 will help you remember the places in your body where tension is most likely to accumulate.

Try to remember also whether there are particular tasks that seem to make your muscles ache. Do they occur at any particular time of the day?

MANAGING STRESS

Stress can be managed in three ways:

- going to a qualified professional for counseling
- restructuring your environment to make it less stressful
- learning relaxation techniques

Going to a Qualified Counselor

This can be a real help for those who feel they need it and have the resources. But since this is a self-help book, you will be functioning as your own counselor. You will need to look within and see what areas you would like to change in your life to make it more pleasant. Only a person who is stuck with the need to be a victim will say, "There's nothing I can do." Obviously that isn't you, or you wouldn't be using this book.

Restructuring Your Environment

We all tend to become oblivious to our surroundings at times. We see them, yet we don't see them. If you go through

your day like a robot, simply doing your tasks and endur-
ing discomfort, it's time now to stop and ask yourself what
you can do to improve your life.

Physical Environment. Have you made your work and
home attractive with pictures, plants, or personal accessories?
Surrounding yourself with soothing colors and soft music
helps you deal with stress.

Job. If you dislike your job, try to find another. You might
want to take night courses or weekend seminars to prepare yourself for a different field or job level. Even if you
can only do this slowly, it will give you something positive to
focus on and you'll be learning something that you enjoy.
Discuss problems on the job with your boss to see if you can
make it a more enjoyable experience.

Work more slowly during the times of day when you begin to drag. Pace yourself, knowing when you tend to experience fatigue. Upgrade your energy during this time by
closing your office door or going into your bedroom to listen
to a relaxation tape, do deep breathing or meditate. (The
specific techniques given in the next section take a few minutes
and can increase your energy tremendously.)

Home. In some ways this is the most difficult area of all to
work on because our relations with our spouses, our children
and ourselves are very much based on upbringing. We
tend to internalize the behavior and beliefs of our own families. We receive these messages very early in life and they
are as much a part of us as our arms and legs. A real conflict occurs when what we would like to have as an adult differs
from what we have been taught to have. You may want a
satisfying sexual relationship but if your parents didn't
have one or taught you that it was to be feared, you may set up

your environment so that it doesn't occur. You may fight with your spouse to avoid intimacy, or you may pick a spouse who is not interested in sex. These are just a few of the hundreds of ways that people unconsciously set themselves up for frustration and stress.

If you are extremely uncomfortable with the personal life that you've constructed for yourself, you may need to work with a counselor. On a day-to-day level, however, there are certainly things that you can do to improve your life. Reading psychology books and inspirational texts, listening to tapes and repeating affirmations to replace the negative parental messages that you learned as a child can all help. Your belief system can slowly be programmed toward what will make you happy. A list of suggested books and tapes is on page 231.

When I question patients, many of them seem to recognize what their problems are even if they aren't sure how to solve them. Many people communicate in a way that doesn't work. They either don't state their wishes directly, do so in an aggressive and combative way, or communicate as a victim about to be kicked.

If you know that you have a problem area, it might help to:

- Ask for feedback from the people around you. Ask your spouse or friends. Be open to the feedback. Don't "kill the messenger" by becoming angry or defensive.

- Negotiate your differences. Businesses collapse when bosses and employees don't listen to each other. Your home is no different. You would never think of screaming at your boss unless you wanted to be fired. Why scream at your children or friends? All it does is drain your energy. Bad communication habits cause stress, disrupt your autonomic nervous system, and can be an environmental trigger for PMS. It is necessary to sit down with other people and discuss problems in a way that can bring a positive result. Discussions work when two people give a little and take a little. This way everyone wins.

We would all like to have exactly what we want 100 percent of the time, but that doesn't happen in real life. For example, you may want to go out and socialize at parties on the weekends. Your spouse may want to stay home and watch TV.

The following way of expressing yourself will *not* work:

You: (angry tone of voice): "It's all your fault. You keep me from having any fun. All we ever do is stay at home."

Even if you honestly feel this way, expressing it in an angry way will only bring you an angry response. You won't be listened to. You may have better luck with:

You: (concerned tone of voice): "I'm not happy with our social life. I would like to go out more often and you like to stay at home. How can we work out this problem?"

This can succeed only if you have a mate or friends who are open to discussing matters with you. But at least you will be part of the solution, not part of the problem.

TECHNIQUES FOR RELAXATION

Many people think of relaxation as what we do while we are asleep. We Westerners tend to be very goal-oriented. We hurry through the day trying to complete tasks as fast as possible and then go on to the next ones. There is a continual sense of urgency—"I've got to get it done"—without much regard for how we get there. This tends to speed up the autonomic nervous system responses that lead to stress and tension and can worsen PMS. With the use of relaxation techniques, tasks get done in the same amount of time and the journey is much more enjoyable.

For example, as I write this book I set daily production goals for myself. To meet these goals I can either rush to get the work done as fast as I can or I can work in a leisurely way. When I work in a rushed manner, I become more nervous and tired by the end of the day. My back muscles feel sore from bending over the typewriter. If I work in a leisurely way, I get out of my chair every hour or two and take a break. I stretch my cramped muscles, do some deep breathing exercises, and clear out my mind. The surprise is that I get more work done the second way—and feel a lot more relaxed and energetic by the end of the workday.

For the last few years, I have been teaching these relaxation methods to patients. We go over these exercises at my office or they learn them on their own using books and tapes that I suggest. Almost without exception they come back very enthusiastic about the results. They say that these exercises calm their minds and their bodies. They usually feel happier and more positive about their lives. They also note improvements in their physical health. A calm mind seems to calm the body: the autonomic nervous system slows down and the body chemistry normalizes.

Here are some simple exercises that I have found to be very helpful for women with PMS:

First Step. Find a comfortable position. For many women, this means lying on their backs. You may also do the exercises sitting up. Try to keep your spine as straight as possible.

Your arms and legs should be uncrossed. It is important that your clothes be loose and comfortable.

Second Step. Focus your attention upon the exercises so that distracting thoughts do not interfere with your concentration. Close your eyes and take a few deep breaths, in and out. This will help to remove your thoughts from the problems and tasks of the day and begin to quiet your mind.

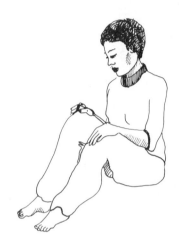

Exercise 1: Concentration

Look at a watch with a second hand. Focus all of your attention upon the hands of the watch. For fifteen seconds don't let any other thoughts enter your mind. At the end of this time, notice your breathing. You will probably find that it has slowed down and is calmer. You may also feel less nervous.

Exercise 2: Deep Abdominal Breathing

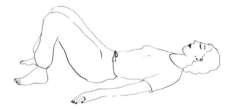

Lie flat on your back with your knees pulled up. Keep your feet slightly apart. Try to breathe in and out through your nose.

Inhale deeply. As you breathe in allow your stomach to relax so that the air flows into your abdomen. Your stomach should balloon out as you breathe in. Visualize the lowest part of your lungs filling up with air.

Imagine that the air you are breathing is filling your body with energy.

Exhale deeply. As you breathe out, imagine the air being pushed out from the bottom of your lungs to the top, as if a tube of toothpaste were being rolled up.

As you exhale, imagine that you are sending love and peace with every breath.

Repeat this sequence until your breathing is slow and regular. Your entire body will feel relaxed. This breathing exercise will also strengthen muscles in your abdomen and chest. It is also very useful for anyone with respiratory problems.

Exercise 3: Discovering Muscle Tension

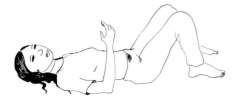

Lie in a comfortable position. Allow your right arm to rest limply, palm down, on the surface next to you.

Now raise just the hand, not the entire arm, and hold it there for fifteen seconds.

How does the top of your forearm feel? Does it feel tight and tense?

Now let your arm drop down and relax. The arm muscles will relax too. They should feel comfortable again.

As you lie there, notice any other parts of your body that carry tension. They will feel tight and a little sore. You may notice a constant dull aching. Tense muscles block blood flow and cut off the supply of nutrients to the tissues. The muscle is poorly oxygenated and in response produces lactic acid.

Exercise 4: Progressive Muscle Relaxation

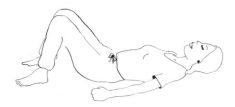

Lie in a comfortable position. Allow your arms to rest limply, palms down, on the surface next to you. Practice your deep breathing from Exercise 2 as you do this exercise.

Clench your hands into fists and hold them tightly for fifteen seconds. As you do this, relax the rest of your body. Then let your hands relax.

Now tense and relax the following parts of your body in this order: your face, shoulders, back, stomach, pelvis, legs, feet, and toes. Hold each part tensed for fifteen seconds and then relax your body for thirty seconds before going on to the next part.

Visualize the tense part contracting, becoming tighter and tighter. On relaxing, see the energy flowing into the entire body like a gentle wave, making all the muscles soft and pliable.

Finish the exercise by shaking your hands and imagining the remaining tension flowing out your fingertips.

This is a particularly useful exercise to do when you feel tension building up during the premenstrual period. It helps to discharge stress in a beneficial way.

Exercise 5: Meditation

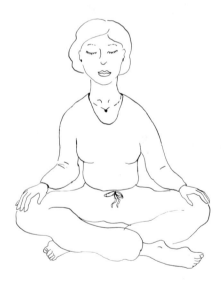

Lie or sit in a very comfortable position.

Close your eyes and breathe deeply. Let your breathing be slow and relaxed.

Focus all of your attention on your breathing. Notice the movement of your chest and abdomen in and out.

Block out all other thoughts, feelings, and sensations. If you feel your attention wandering, bring it back to your breathing.

Say the word IN as you inhale. Say the word OUT as you exhale. Draw out the pronunciation of the word so that it lasts for the entire breath. The word IN sounds like this: i-i-i-i-n-n-n-n-n. The word OUT sounds like this: ow-ow-w-w-w-w-t-t-t-t-t. Repeating these two words will help you to concentrate.

Do this exercise for as long as you are able to, up to five minutes.

This meditation requires you to sit quietly and engage in a simple and repetitive activity. (This can be very difficult at first.) By emptying your mind you give yourself a rest. The metabolism of your body slows down. The brain wave slows from the fast beta wave that predominates during our normal working day to a slower alpha or theta wave. This slower pattern is what appears during sleep or in the period of deep relaxation just prior to falling asleep. Meditating gives your mind a vacation from tension and worry. It is useful to do during the premenstrual period when every little stress is magnified into a monster. After meditating you may wonder what all your upset was about. You will see that situations are not as bad as you believed them to be.

Exercise 6: Affirmations

Sit in a comfortable position. Repeat the following affirmations. Repeat those that are particularly important to you three times.

- My body is strong and healthy.
- My female system is strong and healthy.
- My hormones are balanced and normal.
- My estrogen and progesterone levels are perfectly regulated.
- My body chemistry is balanced and normal.
- I go through my monthly menstrual cycle with ease and comfort.
- I barely know that my body is getting ready to menstruate.
- I feel wonderful each month before I menstruate.
- My mood is calm and relaxed throughout the month.
- I handle stress easily and competently.
- I desire a well-balanced and healthful diet.

• I enjoy eating delicious and nutritious food.
• My body wants food that is high in vitamins and minerals.
• I take time each day to relax and enjoy myself.
• I practice the relaxation methods that I enjoy.

During the time of the month when you are free of premenstrual symptoms, use these affirmations several times a day.

Your state of health is determined by the interaction between your mind and body. It is determined by the thousands of mental messages you send yourself each day with your thoughts. For example, if you do not like yourself, you will be constantly criticizing yourself: the way you look, talk, and act. This will be reflected in your body. Your shoulders will probably slump and your countenance will be lackluster and depressed.

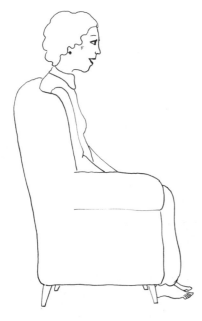

When your body believes that it is sick, it behaves as if it were sick. That is part of the reason that you experience discomfort before your menstrual period. It is not enough to change your nutritional and exercise habits. You also need to change your belief system and the way in which you see your body. This technique of imaging your body the way you want it to be has been used to great benefit for patients with many types of diseases. In his book *Getting Well Again*, Carl Simonton, a cancer radiation therapist, used this technique with his patients. He asked them to imagine that they had strong immune systems capable of fighting a small, puny cancer (instead of the other way around). In a substantial number of cases he saw patients with very serious diseases go into remission.

Exercise 7: Visualizations

Close your eyes. Begin to breathe deeply. Inhale and let this air out slowly. Feel your body begin to relax.

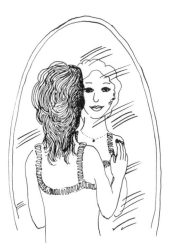

Imagine that the premenstrual period is beginning and to your surprise you feel wonderful. Let a smile come on your face right now and see how good it feels. Let yourself feel happy for a few seconds.

Imagine yourself looking in a mirror. Actually see your body in your mind's eye. You are undressed or wearing a slip or shorts.

You look at your breasts and touch them. To your surprise they feel perfectly normal. They are not tender or swollen.

Look at your abdomen. See it flat and smooth. No bloating has accumulated this month.

Look at your face. It is smooth and relaxed. The smile is still on your face. You feel in command of yourself. You do not feel anxious, irritable, or depressed. Your mood is wonderful. As you look at yourself in the mirror, you know that you can handle any problems that come along, competently and with great ease.

Your complexion is clear and smooth. Touch your face and enjoy how nice it is to have clear skin in the time before your period.

Look at your entire body and enjoy the feeling of energy and optimism that is running through you. You have become very calm.

Now stop visualizing the scene and go back to deep breathing.

You open your eyes and feel very good.

Visualizing this scene should take about forty-five seconds to one minute, perhaps longer if you choose to linger with a particular image. A visualization is successful when it allows you to actually change your feelings about a particular situation.

Your visualization should begin to lay down the mental blueprint for a healthier body and more positive belief system about your health.

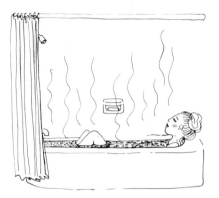

Hot Soak

This is an excellent method to induce relaxation. You can make a mineral bath that is similar to the mineral baths at health spas. Just run a hot tub of water and add one cup of sea salt and one cup of bicarbonate of soda. This is a highly alkaline mixture. It should be used only two to three times during the premenstrual period. It relieves menstrual cramps and helps calm premenstrual anxiety and irritability.

Soak for twenty minutes. You will probably feel very relaxed and sleepy after this bath. It is best taken just before going to sleep at night. Chances are you will sleep very well. You may wake up feeling refreshed and full of energy the next day.

Making the Improvement Permanent

Your state of health is deeply affected by your beliefs. When set in a positive manner, your mind can help to correct imbalances in your hormones and physiology. This chapter has introduced you to many different ways to reset your mind and body. Which exercises you practice will be a matter of your individual taste. Try each one of them at least once. Experiment with them until you find the combination that works for you. Doing all seven will take no longer than fifteen minutes to a half hour, depending on how much time you wish to spend with each one. Ideally the exercises should be done on a daily basis for at least a few minutes a day. Over time, they will help you to gain insight into your negative beliefs and change them into positive new ones. Your ability to cope with stress should be tremendously improved.

DATE _____

Dear Dr. Lark,

☐ I would like to receive further information from the PMS Self-Help Center about your home treatment program.

☐ Please send me information about when your PMS Self-Help Workshop will be in my area.

_____
NAME (PLEASE PRINT)

_____
MAILING ADDRESS

_____
CITY   STATE   ZIP

(____) _____
PHONE   AREA   NUMBER

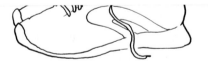

mentioned as
y about aspirin,
as effective.
would go to bed
t wouldn't last
benefits of a well-
l I was in my
le more as my pe-
ed the bene-
ficial effects of exercise in many of my patients.

There are several physiological reasons why exercise relieves PMS. Premenstrual pain causes the breathing to become rapid and shallow. Women also tend to contract their muscles involuntarily when they are in pain or anticipate pain. Both shallow breathing and tight muscles can decrease the amount of blood flow and oxygenation to the tissues. This worsens the congestive symptoms of PMS greatly. Aching in the ankles, feet, and pelvis is often due to fluid retention. (Some women even notice visible swelling in their lower extremities premenstrually.) Exercise corrects all these conditions. The vigorous pumping action of the muscles that occurs with tennis, walking, swimming, and other activities moves blood and other fluids from the congested organs. (Sexual intercourse and orgasm can make you feel better for the same reason.)

Exercise can prevent lower back pain and cramps by strengthening the back and abdominal muscles. Women who exercise regularly often report that their periods are shorter and that they bleed less.

There are also important psychological effects. Exercise reduces premenstrual anxiety and irritability by helping to balance the autonomic nervous system. It gives an effective way to discharge the overactive "fight or flight" pattern that many women experience. Most women note a deep sense of relaxation and peace after they exercise. This may be due to an increased output of endorphins (chemicals made by the brain that have a natural opiate effect and are thought to be the reason for the "runner's high" that many marathoners experience).

Exercise can also improve the posture. Poor posture is another common reason for PMS. Large-breasted women are often self-conscious. They tend to round their shoulders and hunch over to de-emphasize their breast size. This can cause tension across the back and neck. It can also worsen congestion in the breasts by impeding circulation. Many women with PMS have an exaggerated curve of their lumbar spine, which can make low back pain and cramps worse. Dr. Arthur Michele, author of *Orthotherapy* (New York: Evans, 1971), recommends exercising to improve the posture as well as increase the flexibility of the pelvic region. Yoga is particularly good if you have poor posture because it emphasizes slow movement and correct placement of the body.

While moderate and frequent physical activity is beneficial, be aware that a vigorous program of exercise may cause menstrual irregularity. Young women who train for sports competitively or whose careers demand vigorous physical activity often experience a delay in the onset of their menstrual periods. By the age of eighteen, ten percent of ballet dancers are not yet menstruating. Women with normal cycles sometimes menstruate less often or stop entirely if they exercise vigorously. Several reasons have been postulated for this. Ideally, the normal woman has about 22 percent body fat. The athletic woman may have as little as 10 percent. Since estrogen is synthesized by the fatty tissue as well as the ovaries, this can decrease the amount of circulating estrogen. Competitive training can also be emotionally very stressful. It can disrupt the menstrual cycle at the level of the hypothalamus, a part of the brain responsible for triggering the output of pituitary hormones. Most women athletes' cycles resume when their exercise level drops.

Certain types of exercise seem to be better than others for PMS. Walking at a fast pace in fresh air can be particularly beneficial. Try to walk in the early morning sunlight to increase your levels of natural vitamin D. Swimming is excellent for all-around toning and for cardiovascular health. Other enjoyable sports include bicycling, tennis, and moderate jogging.

Try to exercise as often as you can. Some form of exercise every day is preferable for general health. It is very important to increase the level of your activity for a week or two before the onset of your period. Try to exercise before your symptoms start. Don't wait until they reach crisis proportions.

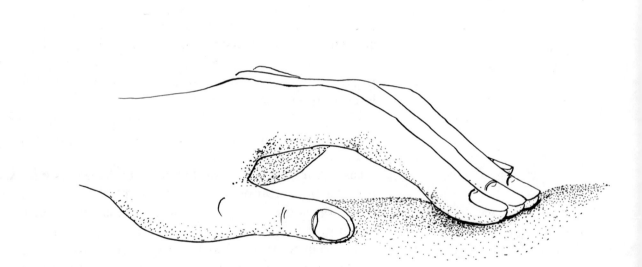

14

Acupressure Massage

Western medicine sees the human body as a series of chemical and mechanical reactions. For example, the heart can fail mechanically as a pump. It can also fail chemically when essential minerals such as calcium and potassium are present in abnormal amounts.

Oriental medicine has traditionally looked at the body in a different way. It is based on the belief that there exists a life energy or "biofield." This life energy is called *chi*. It is different yet similar to electromagnetic energy. Health is thought to occur when the *chi* is equally distributed throughout the body and is present in sufficient amounts. It is thought to energize all the cells and tissues of the body.

This life energy is thought to be distributed throughout the body in channels called meridians. This distribution system is analogous to blood and lymph vessels except that the latter distribute fluid and the meridians distribute a subtle energy. Meridians move energy through the body like invisible rivers. They flow deep into the interior of the body through the organ systems and at times surface on the skin. The place where the energy surfaces on the skin is called the acupuncture point. The electrical resistance of the skin at these points is slightly different from that of the surrounding skin.

Disease is thought to occur when the energy flow through a meridian stops or is blocked. Then the corresponding internal organ system manifests symptoms of disease. The meridian flow can be corrected by stimulating the points on the surface of the skin. These points can be treated either by hand massage, insertion of needles or electrical stimulus. When the normal flow of energy through the body is resumed, the body is believed to heal itself spontaneously.

Stimulation of the acupuncture points can be used to help relieve PMS. The simplest and most effective way is to use finger pressure. This can be done by you or by a friend following simple instructions. It is safe and painless and does not require the use of needles. It can be used without the specialized years of training needed for insertion of needles.

I have used acupressure on my patients in my practice for many problems including pneumonia, viral infections, headaches, and muscle strains, as well as PMS. I have seen acupressure work on stubborn and resistant cases where nothing else seemed to be effective.

HOW TO PERFORM ACUPRESSURE

1. Acupressure should be done either on yourself or by a friend when you are relaxed. Your room should be warm and quiet. Hands should be clean and nails trimmed to avoid bruising yourself. If your hands are cold, put them under warm water.

2. Choose the side of the body to work on that has the most discomfort (for example, your menstrual cramps may be

worse on one side). If both sides are equally uncomfortable, choose whichever one you want. Working on one side seems to relieve the symptoms on both sides. There appears to be a transfer of energy or information from one side to the other.

3. Hold each point indicated in the exercise with a steady pressure for one to three minutes. Pressure should be applied slowly with the tips or balls of the fingers. It is best to place several fingers over the area of the point. If you feel resistance or tension in the area on which you are applying tension, you may want to push a little harder. However, if your hand starts to feel tense or tired, lighten the pressure a bit. Make sure that your hand is comfortable. The acupressure point may feel somewhat tender. This means that the energy pathway or meridian is blocked.

4. During the treatment, the tenderness in the point should slowly go away. You may also have a subjective feeling of energy radiating from this point into the body. Many patients describe this sensation as very pleasant. Don't worry if you don't feel it; not everybody does. The main goal is relief from your PMS.

5. Breathe gently while doing each exercise.

6. The point that you are to hold is shown in the photograph accompanying the text. All of these points correspond to specific points on the acupressure meridians.

7. You may massage the points once a day or more during the time that you have symptoms. You may even want to begin massaging the pressure points a day or two before you anticipate symptoms.

THE EXERCISES

Acupressure Exercise 1: General Balancing of the Energy Pathways

This sequence of points balances the energy flow of the entire body and benefits all of the meridians. It is the most calming of all sequences because it works directly on the spine and the brain. It balances the entire nervous system. It is excellent in helping to relieve the anxiety, mood swings, and irritability that more than 80 percent of women with PMS seem to suffer.

It relieves headaches and is also useful in balancing the energy of the reproductive tract.

——————————1

Sit upright on a chair. Hold each step for 1 to 3 minutes.

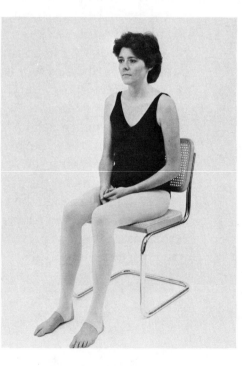

————————2

Left hand holds the point just below the base of the sternum.

    Right hand holds the point 2 inches below the navel.

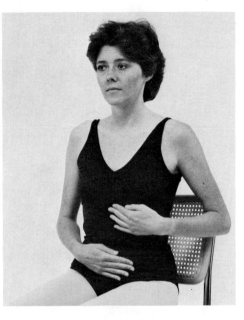

————————3

Left hand does not move.

    Right hand holds the point at the top of the pubic bone.

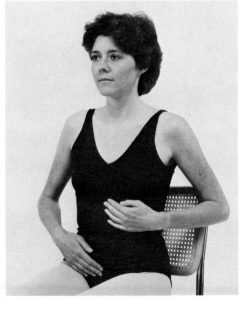

—————————————4

Left hand stays on the point just below the base of the sternum.

Right hand holds the point at the bottom of the tailbone.

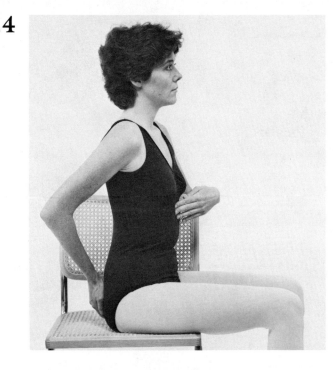

—————————————5

Left hand holds the point below the large vertebra (bone) at the base of the neck.

Right hand is placed 1 inch above the waist on the spine.

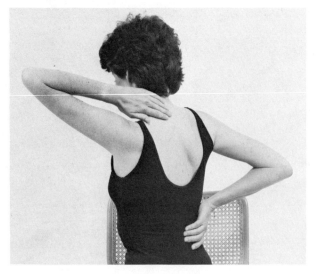

————————6

Left hand holds the point on the spine where it meets the base of the skull.

Right hand stays 1 inch above the waist on the spine.

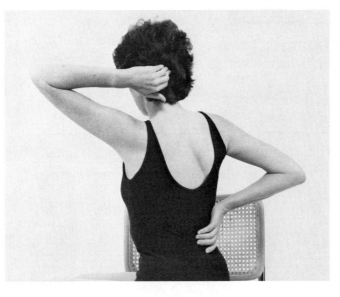

————————7

Left hand moves to the point between the eyebrows.

Right hand holds the point on the top of the head.

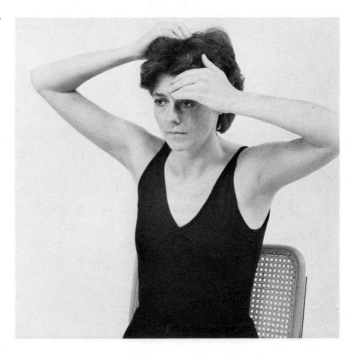

Left hand holds the point between the nipples on the sternum.

Right hand remains at the point on top of the head.

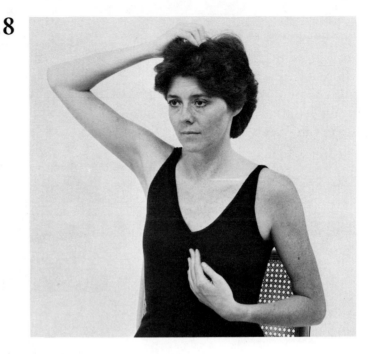

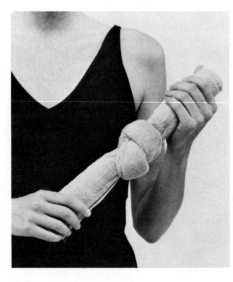

Exercise 2: Balances the Entire Reproductive Tract

This exercise alleviates all menstrual complaints, balances the energy of the female reproductive tract, and relieves low back pain and abdominal discomfort.

Equipment. This exercise uses a knotted hand towel to put pressure on hard-to-reach areas of the back. Place the knotted towel on these points while your two hands are on the other points. This increases your ability to unblock the energy pathways of your body.

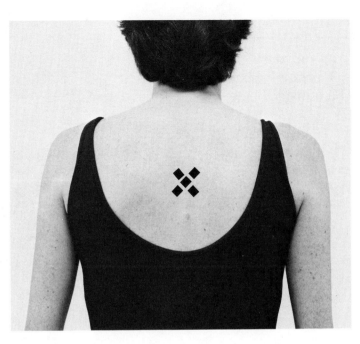

1

Lie on the floor with your knees up. As you lie down, place the towel between the shoulder blades on the spine. Hold each step 1 to 3 minutes.

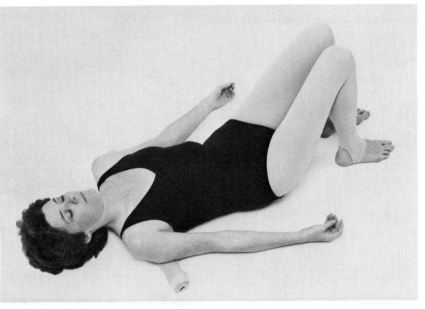

————————2

Cross your arms on your chest. Press your thumbs against the right and left inside upper arms.

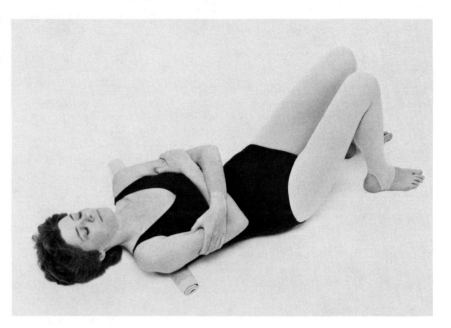

————————3

Left hand holds point at the base of the sternum (breastbone).

Right hand holds point at the base of the head (at the junction of the spine and the skull).

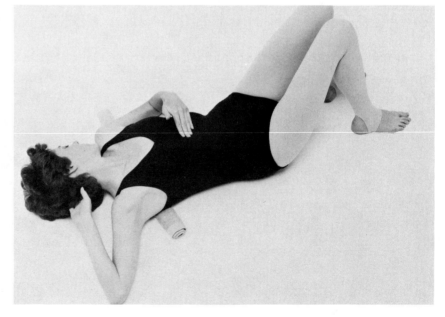

4

Interlace fingers. Place them below your breasts. Fingertips should press directly against the body.

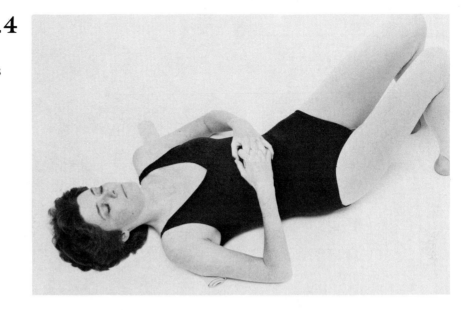

5

Move the knotted towel along the spine to the waistline.

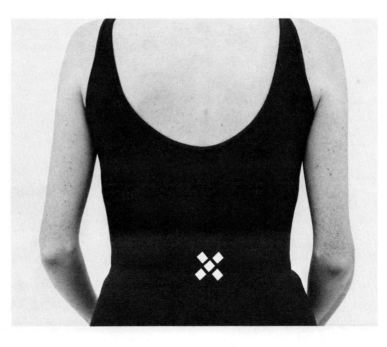

_____ 6

Left hand should be placed
at the top of the pubic bone,
pressing down.
    Right hand holds point
on tailbone.

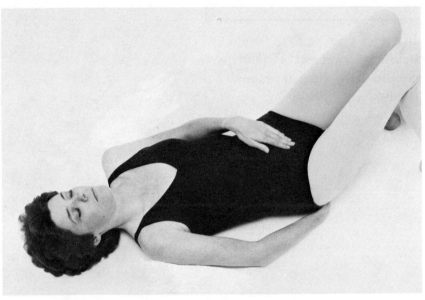

Exercise 3: Relieves Low Back Pain and Cramps

This exercise relieves menstrual cramps and low back
pain by balancing points on the bladder meridian. It also balances the energy of the reproductive organs.

_____ 1

Sit on the floor and prop
your back against a wall or a
heavy piece of furniture.
Hold each step 1 to 3 minutes.
    Alternative Method: Lie
on the floor and put your lower
legs over the seat of a chair.
Follow the exercise from that
position.

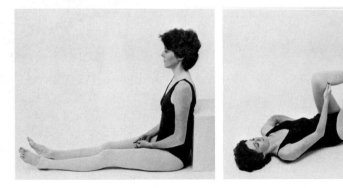

————————2

Place left hand 1 inch above the waist on the muscle to the left side of the spine (muscle will feel firm and ropelike).

Place right hand behind crease of the left knee.

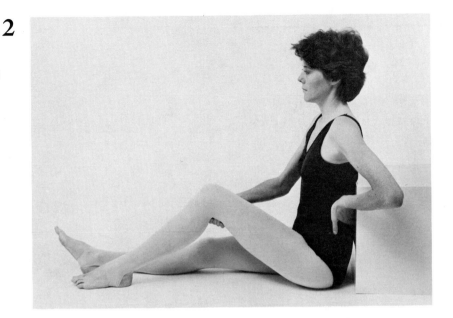

————————3

Left hand stays in the same position.

Right hand is placed on the center of the back of the left calf. This is just below the fullest part of the calf.

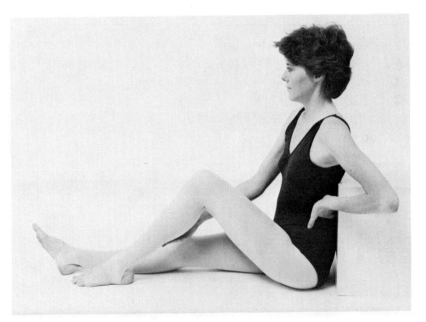

————————————4

Left hand remains 1 inch above the waist on the muscle to the side of the spine.

Right hand is placed just below the ankle bone on the outside of the left heel.

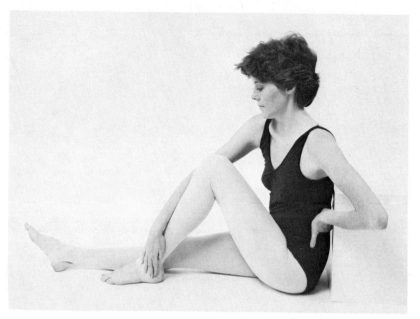

————————————5

Left hand remains 1 inch above the waist on the muscle to the side of the spine.

Right hand holds the front and back of the left little toe at the nail.

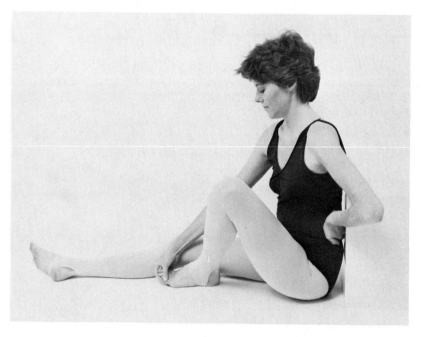

Exercise 4: Relieves Cramps, Bloating, Fluid Retention, Weight Gain

This sequence of points balances the energy flow of the spleen meridian. It is effective for relieving menstrual cramps. It relieves bloating and fluid retention and helps to minimize weight gain in the premenstrual period.

1

Sit up and prop your back against a chair or lie down and put your lower legs on a chair. Hold each step 1 to 3 minutes.

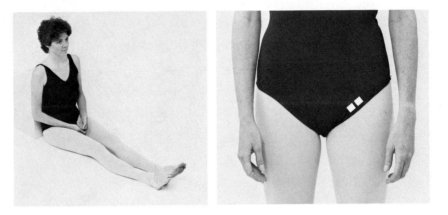

2

Left hand is placed in the crease of the groin where you bend your leg, one-third to one-half way between the hip bone and the outside edge of the pubic bone. Right hand holds a spot 2 to 3 inches above the knee.

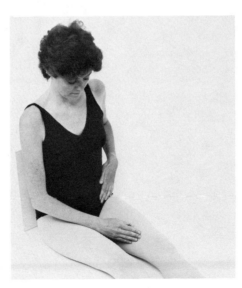

————————3

Left hand remains in the crease of the groin.

Right hand holds point below inner part of knee. To find the point, follow the curve of the bone just below the knee. Hold the underside of the curve with your fingers.

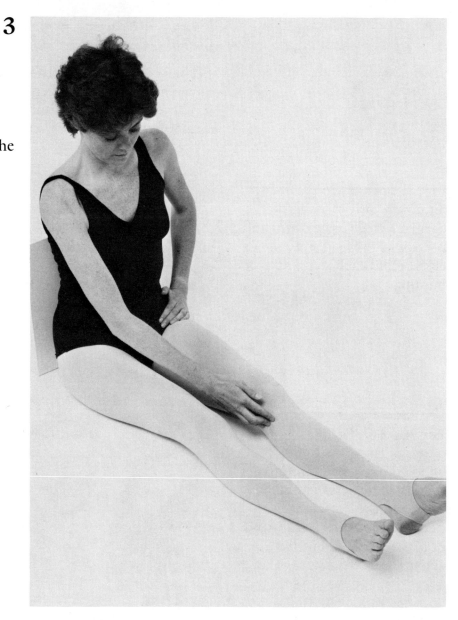

4

Left hand remains in the crease of the groin.

Right hand holds the inside of the shin. To find this point, go four fingerwidths above the ankle bone. The point is just above the top finger.

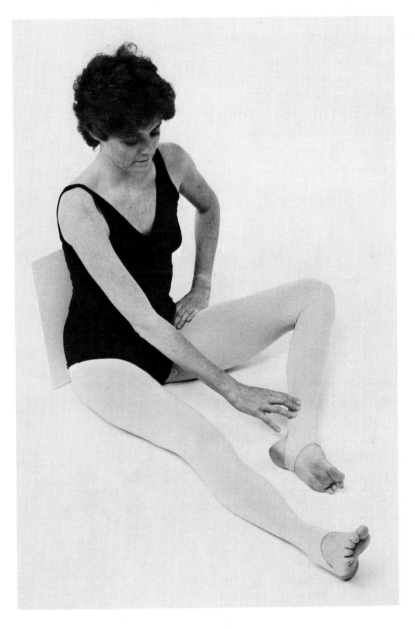

————————5

Left hand remains in the crease of the groin.

Right hand holds the edge of the instep. To find the point, follow the big toe bone up until you hit a knobby, prominent small bone.

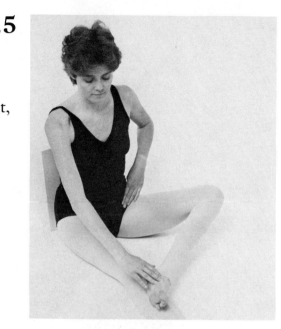

————————6

Left hand remains in the crease of the groin.

Right hand holds the big toe over the nail, front and back of the toe.

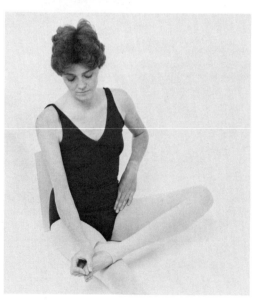

Exercise 5: Relieves Nausea

Relieves premenstrual nausea. This usually occurs in conjunction with cramps and low back pain.

_____1

Lie on the floor or sit up.
Hold 1 to 3 minutes.

_____2

Left index finger is placed in navel and pointed slightly toward the head.

Right hand holds point at the base of the head.

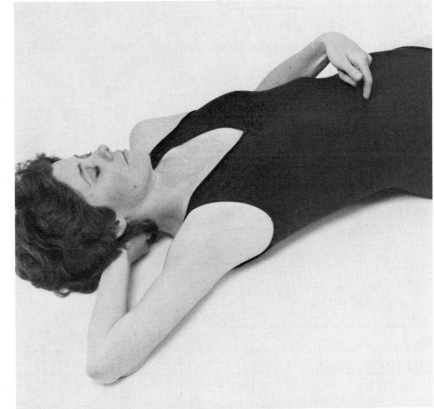

Exercise 6: Relieves Acne

This exercise relieves acne and helps to relieve hives.

———————1

Sit on the floor with the
knees bent. Hold each step 1 to
3 minutes.

———————2

Left hand holds left calf.
   Right hand holds right
calf.

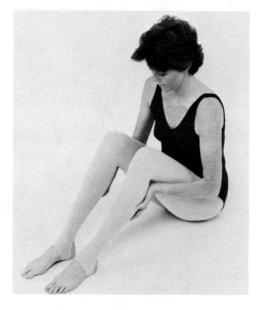

———————3

Cross arms. Left hand holds
right calf.
   Right hand holds left calf.

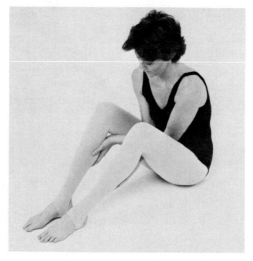

Exercise 7: Relieves Depression, Headaches, Tightness of Neck and Shoulders, and Hypoglycemia

The neck and shoulders generally carry a great deal of tension. Tightness in this area can act as a bottleneck and impede the energy flow of the entire body. Thus the entire body is energized by this exercise. It also relieves depression.

A major treatment point for hypoglycemia is worked on in this exercise. This may help reduce the excessive cravings for sweets that some women notice before their periods.

—————————1

Sit comfortably or lie down. Hold each step 1 to 3 minutes.

—————————2

Left hand holds point at the top of the shoulder blade, 1 to 2 inches to the side of the spine. The point is between the shoulder blade and the spine. It may feel firm and resistant.

Right hand holds the same point on the right side.

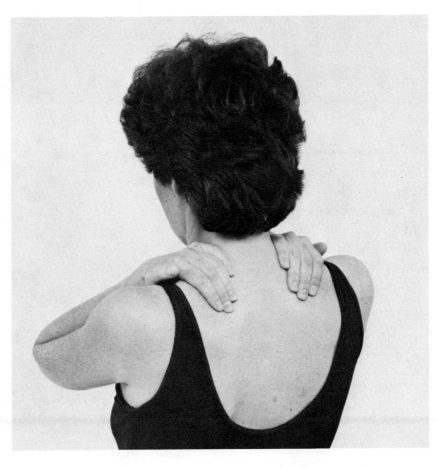

3

Left hand holds points slightly to the back of the top of the shoulder where the neck meets the shoulder.

Right hand holds the same point on the right side.

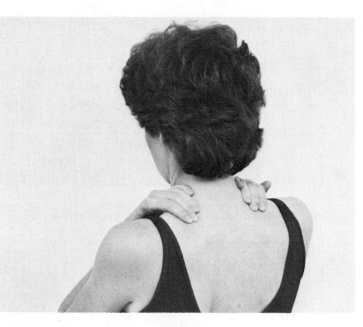

4

Left hand holds the point halfway up the neck, fingers sit on the muscle next to the spine.

Right hand holds the same point on the right side.

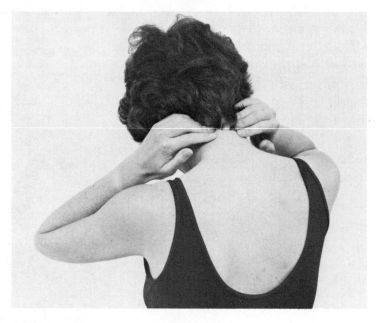

5

Left hand holds the point at the base of the skull 1 to 2 inches out from the spine.

Right hand holds the same point on the right side.

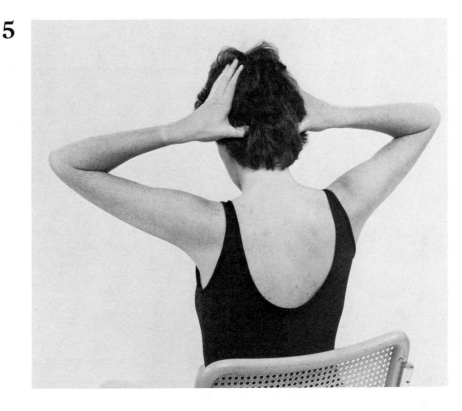

THE RIGHT EXERCISE FOR YOUR SYMPTOMS

The preceding exercises may be useful for each category of PMS. While all of the exercises listed for each symptom group in the chart on page 60 and in the abbreviated chart below can be helpful, the most important exercise for each symptom is the one that has been starred. If you are short of time, you may want to try the starred exercises first. At the beginning, try all the ones that pertain to your symptoms. You may find that you enjoy certain ones more than others. It is only by trial and error that you will find the ones that bring you the most relief.

ACUPRESSURE EXERCISES FOR PREMENSTRUAL SYMPTOMS

Type	Symptoms	Acupressure Exercise
Type A	anxiety, irritability, mood swings	1*, 2
Type C	sugar craving, fatigue, headache	1, 2, 7*
Type H	bloating, weight gain, breast tenderness	1, 2, 4*
Type D	depression, confusion, memory loss	2, 7*
Acne	pimples, oily skin, oily hair	1, 2, 6*
Dysmenorrhea	cramps, low back pain, nausea, vomiting	1, 2, 3*, 4*, 5*

*These exercises are particularly effective.

This chapter was prepared with the help of Marcia Nelson, codirector of the BioCentrics Institute. For information about her classes, contact the BioCentrics Institute, 650 Castro Street, Room 5, Mountain View, CA 94041.

For further information about Jin Shin Do acupressure, you may want to refer to *Jin Shin Do: Acupressure Way of Health* (Japan Publications, distributed by Harper and Row, New York, 1978, $11.50).

Information and self-help charts are also available from the Jin Shin Do Foundation (P.O. Box 1800, Idyllwild, CA 92349), which serves as a referral source for practitioners and teachers throughout Europe and the United States.

15

Massage of the Neurolymphatic and Neurovascular Systems

THE NEUROLYMPHATIC MASSAGE POINTS

The lymphatic system consists of tiny vessels that lead from the periphery of the body to the neck region. From there they empty into the veins leading to the heart. The lymphatics act as a drainage system, gathering up waste products from cells, dead white blood cells, bacteria, and other debris. Once the debris is moved from the lymphatics to the bloodstream, it is processed and excreted from the body. The lymph fluid moves through its channels by mild contractions of the lymph ducts and the surrounding skeletal muscles.

If a person overburdens the lymph system by eating improperly or not exercising, lymphatic fluid can accumulate and cause congestion in a particular area of the body. This was first noted by Dr. Frank Chapman, an osteopath who practiced in the early part of this century. He found that when the energy flow to the lymphatic system is blocked, reflex points regulating the flow of lymph turn off, shutting down the overburdened system like circuit breakers. These reflex points are located primarily on the back and chest. They are small and grainy in texture, usually no larger than a pea, and can be felt over a muscle group.

When there are blocks, pain and congestion appear in that area. Chapman found that this correlated to organ-system and endocrine dysfunction. Firm rubbing of these points can decrease the symptoms significantly. You may want to try massaging these points, especially if the acupressure points don't work. If lymphatic congestion is the cause, pain should decrease over a few days. Locate the points on your body as indicated by the following photographs. Massage deeply and firmly with the fingers for twenty to thirty seconds.

Neurolymphatic Point 1: Relieves Anxiety, Mood Swings, Irritability, Depression, Breast Tenderness, and Bloating

Massage each area shown in the photographs for 20 to 30 seconds.

Front of the body: Area is located between the fifth and sixth ribs, extending from the nipple to the breastbone on the right and left sides.

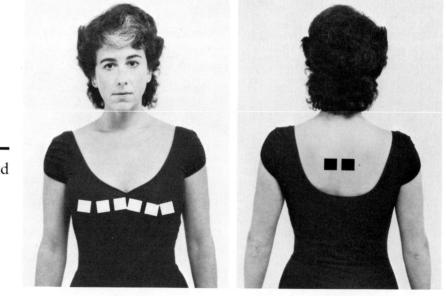

Back of the body: Area is located one inch to either side of the spine (at the levels of the fifth, sixth, and seventh thoracic vertebrae). Look for the soft area between the bones and then move 1 inch to the side.

Neurolymphatic Point 2: Relieves Fluid Retention, Weight Gain and Acne

Massage each area shown in the photographs for 20 to 30 seconds.

Front of the body: Area is located 1 inch up from the navel, 1 inch to either side.

Back of the body: Area is located 1 inch to either side of the spine (between the twelfth thoracic and the first lumbar vertebrae). This is just below the level of the last ribs.

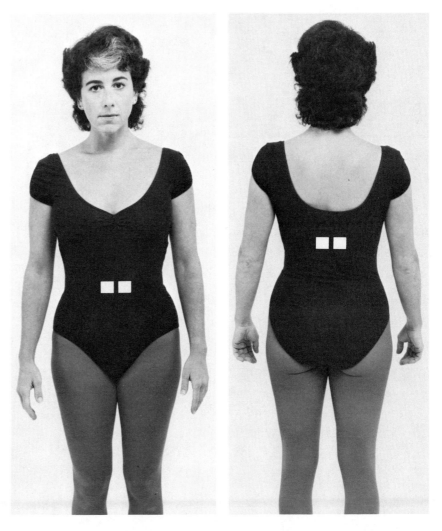

Neurolymphatic Point 3: Use for Carbohydrate Craving, Dizziness, Fatigue

Massage each area shown in the photographs for 20 to 30 seconds.

Front of the body: Area is located 2 inches above the navel and an inch to either side.

Back of the body: Area is located 1 inch to either side of the spine at the level of the last ribs. (This is between the tenth and eleventh thoracic vertebrae and the eleventh and twelfth thoracic vertebrae.)

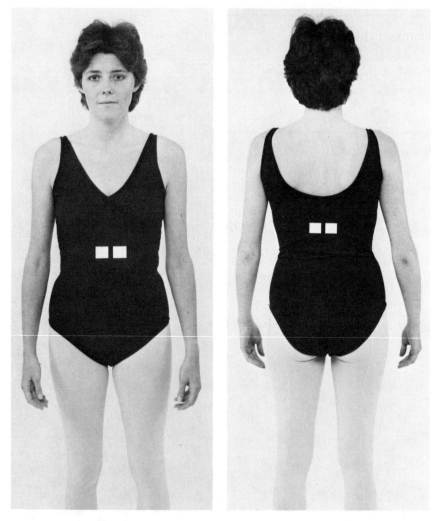

Neurolymphatic Point 4: Use for Carbohydrate Craving, Dizziness, Fatigue

Massage each area shown in the photographs for 20 to 30 seconds.

Front of the body: On the left side of the chest between the seventh and eighth ribs, 1 to 2 inches to the side of the midline.

Back of the body: One inch to either side of the spine (between the seventh and eighth thoracic vertebrae).

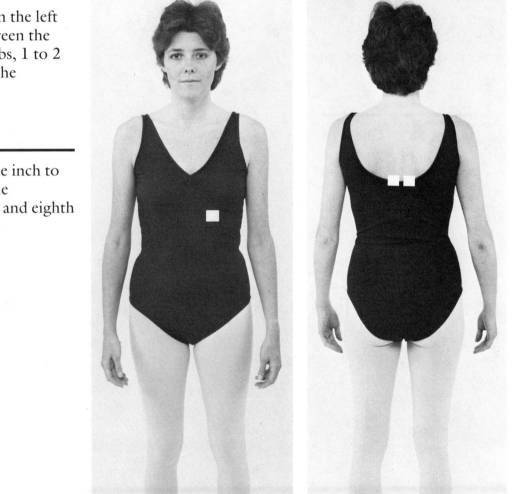

Neurolymphatic Point 5: Relieves Cramps, Low Back Pain.

Massage each area shown in the photographs for 20 to 30 seconds.

Front of the body: Points are located at the upper and inner edges of the pubic bone.

Back of the body: One inch to either side of the spine (at the upper edge of the second lumbar vertebra).

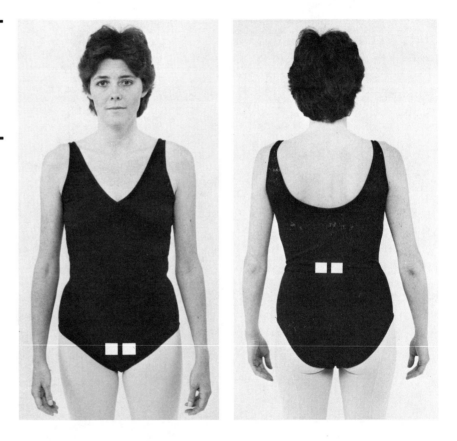

THE NEUROVASCULAR HOLDING POINTS

The neurovascular holding points were discovered by Terrence Bennett, a pioneer in the field of chiropractic. He found that stimulating skin areas with light touch could

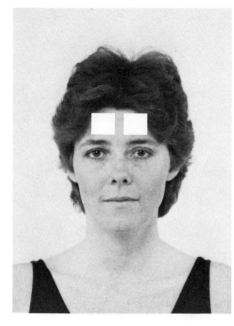

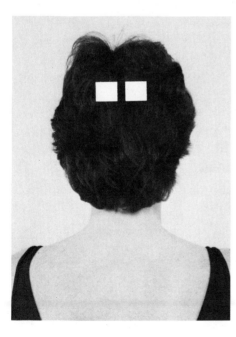

improve blood circulation in deep organ systems. He observed these changes in many patients by watching their organs through a fluoroscope while pressure was being applied to their skin.

Neurovascular points are located mainly on the head. They should be touched lightly with the pads of the fingers. After holding the points for a few seconds, a slight pulsation will be felt. This pulse is not related to the heartbeat. It is thought to be the pulsation of the microcapillary bed in the skin. These points can be held from twenty seconds to five minutes, depending on the severity of the problem. For PMS, their greatest use is in treating symptoms related to emotional upset.

Neurovascular Point 1: Relieves Anxiety, Mood Swings, Irritability, Depression, and Tension Headaches

Points can be held up to five minutes. Concentrate on whatever feelings or situations are upsetting you. Try to feel your upset as strongly as you can. After a time, you will find that you have difficulty concentrating on the problem. It will seem to fade and you may feel much more peaceful at the end of the exercise. This is the most important exercise for relieving emotional upsets.

Frontal eminence: Located on the forehead between the eyebrows and the hairline.

Neurovascular Point 2: Relieves Anxiety, Mood Swings, Irritability, Depression, and Fatigue

Point can be held up to five minutes. Hold until negative emotion fades and energy improves.

Parietal fontanel: located at the back of the head in the midline. This corresponds to the soft spot on the back of a baby's head.

THE RIGHT POINTS FOR YOUR SYMPTOMS

The most important neurolymphatic massage points and neurovascular holding points for you are those listed next to your symptoms on the chart.

NEUROLYMPHATIC AND NEUROVASCULAR POINTS FOR PREMENSTRUAL SYMPTOMS

Type of PMS	Symptoms	Neurolymphatic (NL) and Neurovascular (NV) Points
Type A	anxiety, irritabil-ity, mood swings	NL-1, NV-1, NV-2
Type C	sugar craving, fa-tigue, dizziness, headache	NL-3, NL-4, NV-2
Type H	bloating, weight gain, breast tenderness	NL-1, NL-2
Type D	depression, confu-sion, memory loss, insomnia	NL-1, NV-1, NV-2
Acne	pimples, oily skin, oily hair	NL-2
Dysmenorrhea	cramps, low back pain, nausea, vomiting	NL-5

16

Yoga for PMS

Yoga classes can be found almost everywhere—on television, at your local YWCA and community centers, and at yoga institutes. It is as American as the hamburger or pizza, yet it originated thousands of years ago in India. It was first recorded and systematized in the third century B.C. by the Indian sage Patanjali. His work constitutes an important part of orthodox Indian philosophy. His commentaries are still widely studied and form the basis for yoga as it is practiced today.

The traditional goal of yoga has been to promote balance and harmony in the practitioner. Done properly, the exercises promote health on all levels—physical, mental, emotional, and spiritual.

There are numerous systems of yoga, each providing health through different methods of physical and mental exercises. This chapter deals with the practice of hatha yoga, the type most commonly taught in the United States. Hatha yoga is based on physical exercises called *asanas* and breathing exercises called *pranayama*. It is important that you focus and concentrate on the postures. First your mind visualizes how the exercise is to look and then your body follows with the correct placement of the pose. The exercises are done through slow, controlled stretching movements. This slowness allows you to have greater control over your body movements. You minimize the possibility of injury and maximize the benefit to the particular part of the body that your attention is being directed toward.

HOW TO PERFORM YOGA FOR PMS

1. Yoga should be performed in a relaxed and unhurried manner. Be sure to set aside adequate time, between ten to thirty minutes, so that you do not feel rushed. Your work area should be quiet, peaceful, and uncluttered.

2. Choose a flat area and work on a mat or a blanket. This will make you more comfortable while you do the exercises.

3. Wear loose, comfortable clothing. It is better that you work without socks to give your feet complete freedom of movement and to prevent slipping.

4. Evacuate your bowels or bladder before you begin the exercises. Wait at least two hours after eating to exercise.

5. Try to practice these movements on a regular basis. Every day for a few minutes is best, particularly when you have PMS. If that is not possible, then try to practice them every other day.

6. Pay close attention to the initial instructions when beginning an exercise. Look at the placement of the body as shown in the photographs. This is very important, for if the pose is practiced properly, you are much more likely to have relief of your PMS.

7. Try to visualize the pose in your mind, then follow with proper placement of the body.

8. Move slowly through the pose. This will help promote flexibility of the muscles and prevent injury.

9. Follow the breathing instructions provided in the exercise. Most important, do not hold your breath. Always allow your breathing to flow. It is important that you time your breathing with the placement of the body position.

10. Always rest for a few minutes after doing yoga stretches.

11. Don't be discouraged if you can't do as much as the model in these photos.

WARM-UPS

These exercises should be done the first week or two of your program. Warm-ups promote flexibility and mobility throughout the body. They will prepare you for the specific exercises you will be using to help correct PMS. Try each warm-up exercise at least once. Then put together your own routine. You may find that you want to do all six of them on a regular basis or perhaps only a few. Warm-ups should always precede the PMS corrective exercises.

Stretch 1: Chest Expander

This exercise improves circulation to the upper half of the body and energizes and stimulates it. It also loosens and stretches tense muscles in the upper body, especially the shoulders and back, and expands the lungs.

1

Stand easily. Arms should be at your sides, feet are hip distance apart.

2

Extend your arms forward until your palms touch.

3

Bring your arms back slowly and gracefully until you can clasp them behind your back. Exhale, then straighten your clasped hands and arms as far as you can without discomfort. Remember to stand upright; body should not bend forward. Breathe deeply into the chest.

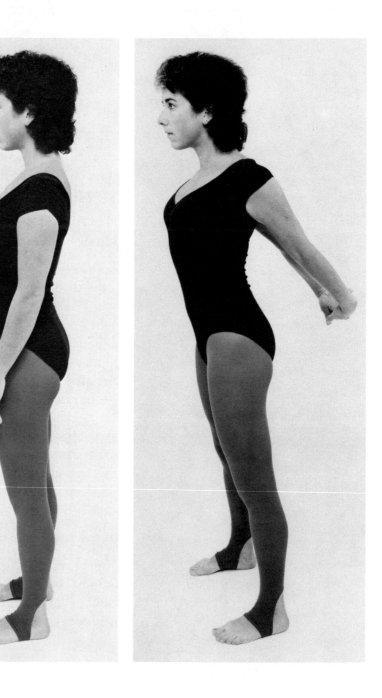

4

Inhale deeply and bend backward from the waist. Keep your hands clasped and your arms held high. Drop your head backward a few inches and look upward as you relax your shoulders and the back of your neck. Hold this position for a few seconds.

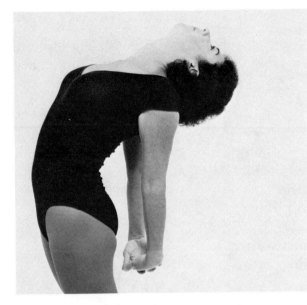

5

As you hold your breath, bend forward at the waist, bringing your clasped hands and arms up over your back. Relax your neck muscles and keep your knees straight. Hold for a few seconds.

6

Exhale as you return to the upright position. Unclasp your hands and allow your arms to rest easily at your sides. Repeat entire sequence 3 times.

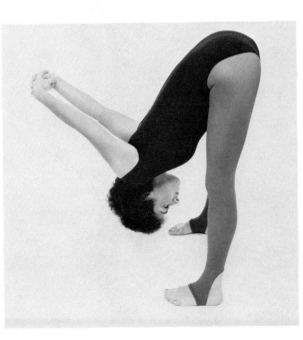

Stretch 2: Arm and Leg Stretch

This exercise relieves tension in the hips and shoulders, strengthens the legs and back, and aids in balance.

———————1

Stand easily with your arms at your sides.

Raise your right arm slowly overhead. Shift your weight to your right leg.

Catch your left ankle with your left hand, bending leg at the knee. You will be balancing yourself on your right leg.

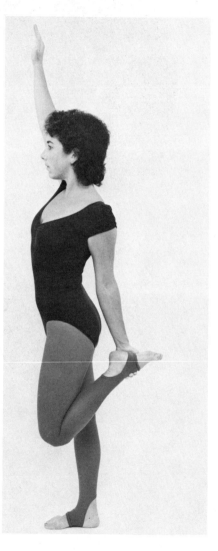

Gently stretch your back by bringing your right hand back a few inches and pulling your left leg up a few inches and moving it away from your body. This should be done slowly. The left arm remains straight to open the shoulder.

Slowly return to your original resting position.

Repeat exercise on opposite foot.

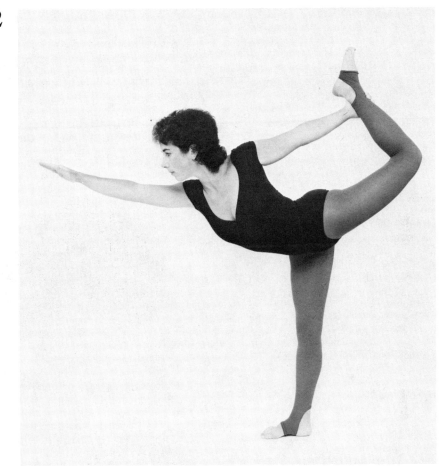

Stretch 3: Neck Rolls

This exercise relieves stiffness and tension in the neck, lubricates the vertebrae, and strengthens the muscles of the neck. You may want to repeat this exercise several times a day if your neck is particularly stiff. You may hear a gritty sound at first. This can accompany stiff and contracted muscles. Visualize your neck rolling slowly and smoothly on ball bearings as you do this exercise.

—————————1

Sit in a chair with your arms and shoulders relaxed. First breathe in deeply, then exhale and allow your head to come all the way forward on to your chest, keeping the spine straight. Hold for a few breaths.

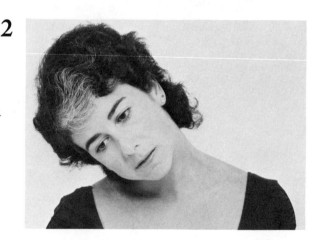

—————————2

Exhale and bring your right ear to the right shoulder, keeping the right shoulder completely relaxed. Hold for a few breaths.

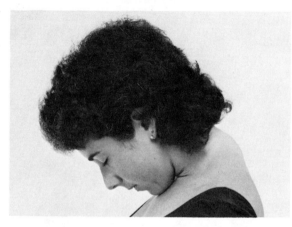

————————3

Exhale and allow your head
to drop back, keeping the spine
straight and the shoulders
relaxed. Hold for a few breaths.

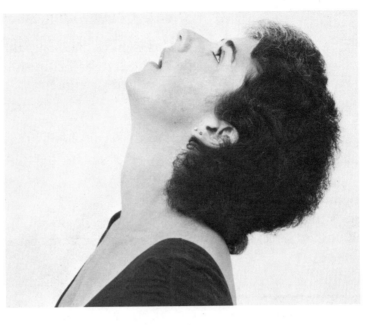

————————4

Bring your left ear to the left
shoulder, keeping your left
shoulder relaxed. Hold for a
few breaths.
   Bring your head to the
original position, keeping your
chin forward. Slowly repeat
the exercise moving in the
opposite direction.

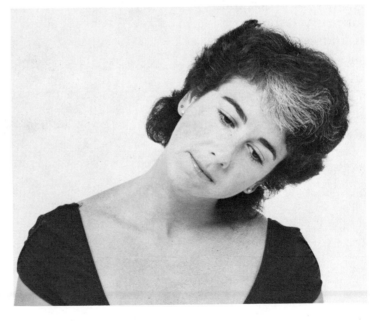

Stretch 4: Rock and Roll

This exercise massages the entire neck and spine and flexes the vertebral column. It will invigorate and energize you, reducing fatigue.

———1

Lie on your back. Bend and raise your knees to your chest, clasping them with your hands. Hands should be interlocked behind knees.

———2

Raise your head toward your knees and gently rock back and forth on your curved spine. Note the roundness of your back and shoulders. Keep the chin tucked in as your roll back. Avoid rolling back too far on your neck.

Rock back and forth 5 to 10 times.

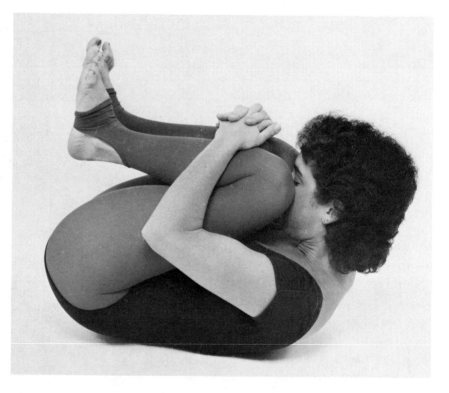

Stretch 5: The Pump

This exercise strengthens the back and abdominal muscles, improves blood circulation through the pelvis, and calms anxiety and nervousness.

————————1

Lie down and press the small of your back into the floor. This permits you to use your abdominal muscles without straining your lower back.

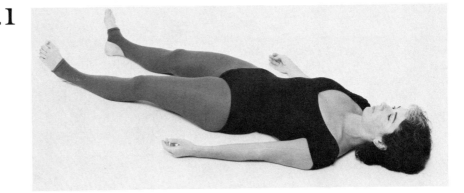

————————2

Raise your right leg slowly while breathing in. Keep your back flat on the floor and let the rest of your body remain relaxed. Move your leg very slowly; imagine your leg being pulled up smoothly by a spring. Do not move your leg in a jerking manner. Hold for a few breaths.

Lower your leg and breathe out.

Repeat the same exercise on your left side. Then alternate legs, repeating the exercise 5 to 10 times.

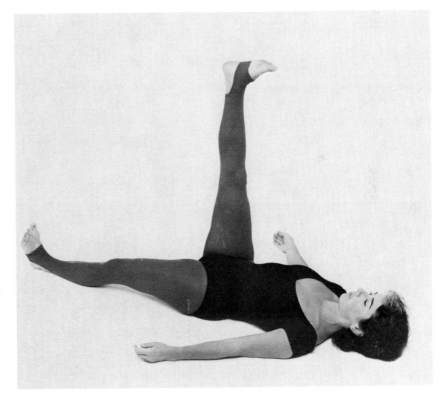

Stretch 6: Spinal Flex

This exercise emphasizes freer pelvic movement with controlled breathing, energizes and rejuvenates the female reproductive tract, and tones the abdominal organs (pancreas, liver, and adrenals). It may also help relieve premenstrual carbohydrate craving and dizziness. It may even help to relieve premenstrual acne.

1

Lie on your back with your knees bent and your feet on the floor close to your buttocks.

2

Exhale and press the lower back into the floor, raising the buttocks slightly.

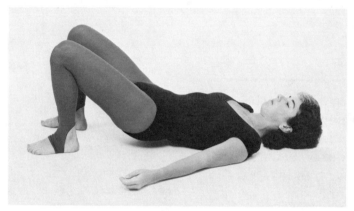

3

Arch the back slightly.

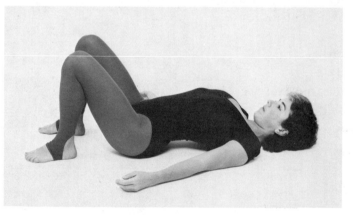

4

Inhale and lift your lower back off the floor. This stretches the region from the sternum to the pelvis.

Repeat this exercise 10 times. Always lift your navel up on the in-breath. Always elongate your spine and press the lower back down on the out-breath.

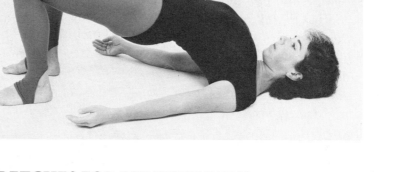

STRETCHES FOR RELIEVING PMS

These exercises should be done after mastering the warm-ups. You may want to start these on week 2 of your program (or week 3 if you prefer to pace yourself a little slower). These exercises energize the entire female tract and relieve low back problems. They also relieve specific symptoms of PMS.

Stretch 7: Upward-Facing Dog

This exercise relieves low back pain and strengthens the spine. It improves blood circulation to the pelvic region and encourages chest expansion and lung elasticity. It also elevates mood and can help to relieve depression.

1

Lie on the floor on your stomach, head facing downward. Place your palms on the floor under your shoulders, fingers pointing straight ahead.

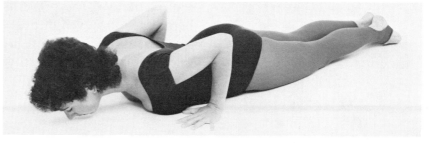

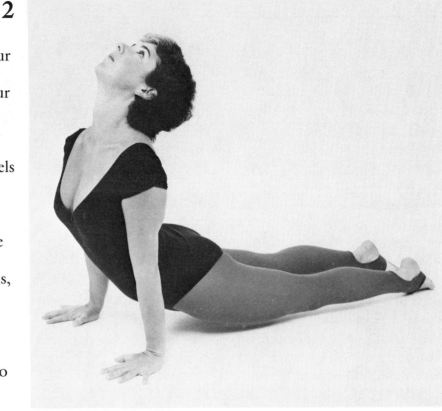

As you inhale, raise your head and trunk, stretching your spine forward and curving it into a gentle C. Make sure your elbows are straight. Avoid hunching up your shoulders. Hips and knees lift off the floor. Legs are straight and heels press back to help stretch the spine. The weight of the body will rest only on the hands and toes. Hold the pose 30 seconds to 1 minute, breathing deeply. Spine, thighs, and calves should be fully stretched and the buttocks contracted.

Bend your elbows, releasing the stretch. Return to the original position and rest for a minute.

Stretch 8: The Locust

This exercise strengthens the lower back, abdomen, buttocks, and legs, and prevents low back pain and cramps. It helps to reduce weight in the thighs and hips and tighten and firm the skin in these areas. It also energizes the entire female reproductive tract, thyroid, liver, intestines, and kidneys.

1

Lie face down on the floor. Make fists with both your hands and place them under your hips. This prevents compression of the lumbar spine while doing the exercise.

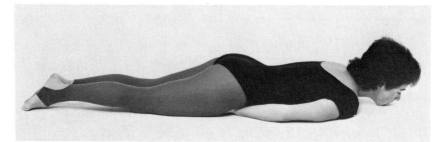

2

Straighten your body and raise your right leg with an upward thrust as high as you can keeping your hips on your fists. Hold for 5 to 20 seconds if possible.

Lower the leg and slowly return to your original position. Repeat on the left side, then with both legs together. Remember to keep your hips resting on your fists.

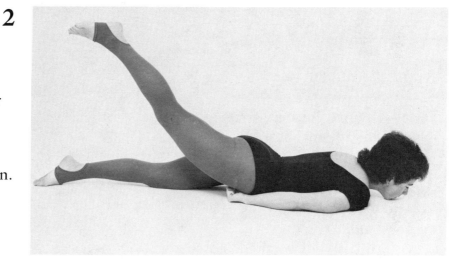

Stretch 9: The Bow

This exercise stretches the entire spine and helps to relieve low back pain and cramps. It stretches the abdominal muscles and strengthens the back, hips, and thighs. It also stimulates the digestive organs and endocrine glands. It may help to relieve sugar craving, oily skin and acne. And, finally, it relieves depression, fatigue, and lethargy, improving your energy and elevating your mood.

1

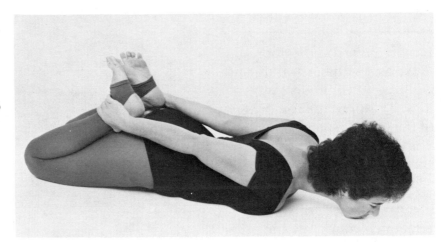

Lie face down on the floor, arms at your sides.

Slowly bend your legs at the knees and bring your feet up toward your buttocks. Reach back with your arms and carefully take hold of first one foot and then the other. Flex your feet to make grasping them easier.

2

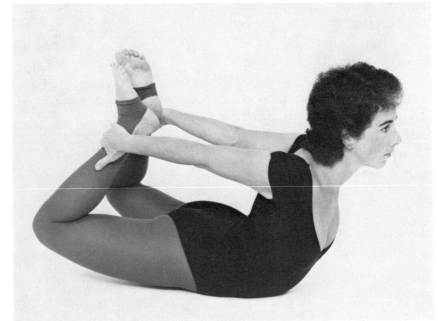

Inhale and raise your trunk from the floor as far as possible. Lift your head and bring your knees as close together and as close to the floor as possible. Squeeze the buttocks. Imagine your body looking like a gently curved bow. Hold for 10 to 15 seconds. Tying your knees together with a soft tie may help you do this exercise.

Slowly release the posture. Allow your chin to touch the floor and finally release your feet and return them slowly to the floor. Return to your original position.

Stretch 10: Child's Pose

This exercise gently stretches the lower back. It is excellent for calming anxiety and irritability. It also relieves menstrual cramps.

——————— 1

Sit on your heels. Bring your forehead to the floor, stretching the spine as far as over your head as possible. Close your eyes. Hold for as long as this is comfortable.

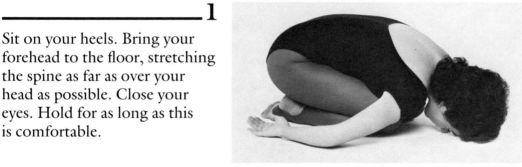

Stretch 11: Wide-Angle Pose

This exercise opens the entire pelvic region, energizes the female reproductive tract, and relieves bloating and fluid retention in legs and feet.

——————— 1

Lie on your back, with your legs against the wall and extended out like a V or an arc and your arms extended to the side. Hips should be as close to the wall as possible, buttocks on the floor. Legs should be spread apart as far as they can and still remain comfortable. Breathing easily, hold for 1 minute, allowing the inner thighs to relax.

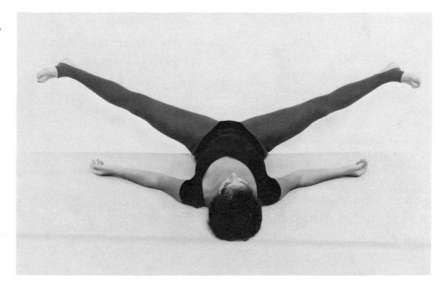

————————2

Bring legs together and hold for 1 minute.

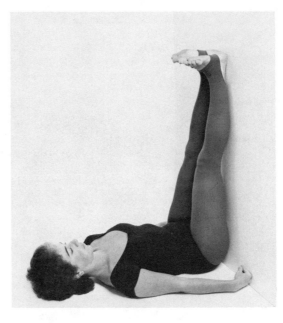

Stretch 12: The Plow

This exercise improves the elasticity of the spine, strengthens the back and relaxes the abdomen and neck. It helps to reduce weight in the hips, thighs, legs, and abdomen. It improves circulation to the brain. It also reduces swelling and fluid retention in the legs and ankles.

————————1

Put a chair on your mat. Lie on your back, facing upward, away from the chair. Arms are at your sides and palms are facing downward so that they press against the floor. Legs should be together.

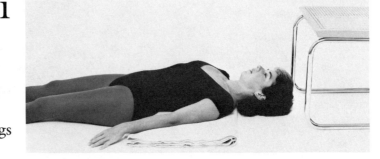

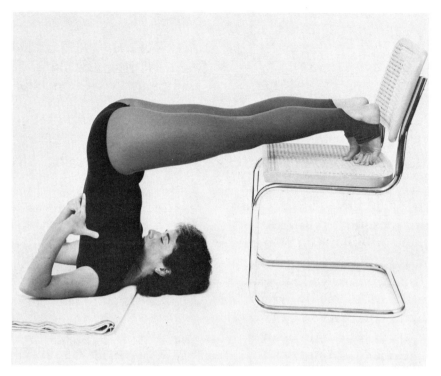

2

Slowly raise your legs and hips over your head until your toes touch the chair. This should be done without jerking, so bend your knees if necessary. (This exercise is usually done by bringing the legs and hips over the head until the toes touch the floor, but bringing the feet all the way to the floor could be harmful for women with PMS, since they often have a concavity of the back.) Lift the spine by stretching the back muscles as much as possible. This exercise will alleviate compression of the lumbar spine.

To come out of this posture, bend your knees and roll down slowly onto your back. Return to your original position.

Stretch 13: The Sponge

This exercise relieves anxiety and irritability and reduces eye tension and swelling of the face. It relieves menstrual cramps and low back pain if a rolled towel is placed under the knees.

1

Lie on your back. Your arms should be at your sides, palms up. Close your eyes and relax your whole body. Inhale slowly, breathing from the diaphragm. As you inhale, visualize the energy in the air around you being drawn in through your entire body. Imagine that your body is porous and open like a sponge so that this energy can be drawn in and revitalize every cell of your body. Exhale slowly and deeply, allowing every ounce of tension to be drained from your body.

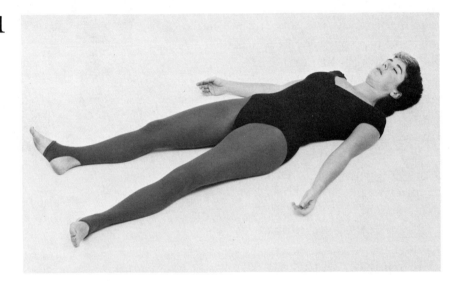

THE RIGHT STRETCH FOR YOUR SYMPTOMS

The preceding exercises may be useful for each category of PMS. Prior to doing the specific correctives, it is recommended that you spend the first week or two of your program doing the warm-up exercises. They are meant to tone and improve flexibility of your entire body. Determine which warm-ups you enjoy the most and practice them on a regular basis, either daily or every other day.

Beginning on week 2 or 3, they can be followed by the specific correctives for PMS. For your convenience the exercises are listed here according to the symptoms they relieve.

- *Type A* (anxiety, irritability, mood swings):
  Pump, Child's Pose, Sponge.

- *Type C* (sugar craving, fatigue, headaches):
  Spinal Flex, Bow.

- *Type H* (bloating, weight gain, breast tenderness):
  Wide Angle Pose, Plow, Sponge.

- *Type D* (depression, confusion, memory loss):
  Upward Facing Dog, Bow.

- *Acne* (pimples, oily skin and hair):
  Spinal Flex, Bow.

- *Dysmenorrhea* (cramps, low back pain,
  nausea, and vomiting):
  Arm and Leg Stretch, Pump, Locust, Bow, Child's Pose, Plow, Sponge.

This chapter was prepared with the help of Rose Bank, co-director of the BioCentrics Institute in Mountain View, California. For more information about her classes, contact the BioCentrics Institute, 650 Castro St., Room 5, Mountain View, CA 94041.

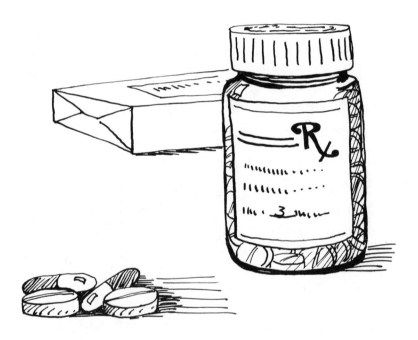

17

Treating PMS with Drugs

Drug treatment of PMS comes last in this book, because this is a self-help book, but if your symptoms of PMS are severe, you may well want to go to your doctor first for the rapid symptomatic relief drugs can offer. Then, by following the self-help program, you should be able to cut back your dosage fairly quickly, and, unless you have a severe case, eventually give up the drug completely.

There have been some wonderful advances in the field of medicine and pharmacology. Treatments are available now for certain PMS symptoms—particularly cramps and mood swings—that simply were not around ten years ago. This is due in part to our increased awareness about the chemical imbalances that cause PMS.

Dysmenorrhea

Particularly noteworthy are the medications that control menstrual cramps or dysmenorrhea. Menstrual cramps are extremely common, occurring in half of all women who menstruate. They can be extremely painful, occurring in the lower back, thighs, and abdomen. Accompanying symptoms include nausea, vomiting, fainting, and diarrhea. The pain normally occurs a few days before or a few days after the onset of menses. In some cases, the pain is caused by fibroid tumors or polyps, which can be found with a simple pelvic exam. But in most cases, "primary dysmenorrhea" is the diagnosis: that is, no physical lesion is found to be causing the pain.

The reason for primary dysmenorrhea was unknown until twenty years ago, when Dr. V. R. Pickles of Sheffield University in England noted a correlation between prostaglandin levels and dysmenorrhea. Prostaglandins are chemicals produced by the lining of the uterus. Their levels increase until menstruation. There are nine groups of prostaglandins that cause either relaxation or contraction of the uterus. Prostaglandin F is primarily responsible for causing uterine contractions, in contrast to prostaglandin E which causes relaxation. If excess prostaglandin is produced or if there is an excess of F over E, the uterus contracts too actively, causing cramping and pain.

Through the research work of doctors such as Dr. Pickles and Dr. Penny Wise Budoff, a Long Island gynecologist, drugs used in treating inflammatory diseases like arthritis were found to inhibit both prostaglandin synthesis and activity. These drugs include Indocin, Motrin, and Ponstel. These medications have been approved by the FDA for the treatment of menstrual pain and are being used widely today. Although these drugs are generally considered to be safe, they can have serious side effects and, like most drugs, require careful monitoring by doctor and patient.

More controversial is the use of progesterone. Eighty percent of women with premenstrual tension note significant mood swings, irritability, and anxiety. These can occur for a few days to as much as several weeks out of the month. As far back as the 1930s these mood swings were thought to be due to hormonal imbalance—specifically, estrogen excess in the face of relative progesterone deficiency. Katharina

Dalton, an English gynecologist, began treating women with progesterone thirty years ago. Her work was not generally accepted, and she was a lone voice advocating the use of progesterone for many years. This is still considered a controversial question, chiefly because some English researchers have tried to replicate Dalton's studies without success.

The use of natural (soy, yam, or animal derived) progesterone has not yet been approved in this country by the FDA. There are very few physicians who currently use it, partly because the FDA requires that physicians using progesterone must ask their patients to sign an informed consent. This means that the patient has been notified of the potential risks as well as the legal status of the hormone.

Nevertheless, I have been using progesterone for the last few years in my medical practice, and have found it to have fewer side effects than the more commonly used drugs. I use a form of progesterone derived from soybeans that I obtain from a pharmacy in Wisconsin. It is currently available as a vaginal cream or a suppository that can be used either rectally or vaginally. This is much more convenient for patients than the original form, which was available only as an injection. I have seen excellent results in most of my patients who use it and strongly advocate its use in appropriate cases. If you are interested in using progesterone, ask your doctor if he or she is familiar with it. Unfortunately, many still are not. You might refer your physician to the work of Dr. Dalton (see bibliography) or to the PMS Action group in Madison, Wisconsin (see page 229). Both are excellent sources of information for physicians as well as women with PMS.

Acne

Mild acne can be treated locally by washing the skin several times a day and using skin scrubs containing benzyl peroxide and salicylic acid. For more serious cases, many doctors prescribe wide-spectrum antibiotics like tetracycline. Vitamin A compounds applied to the skin as a solution or with presoaked swabs have been very useful in treating cystic acne. But the best treatment for acne is the nutritional treatment I described in Chapter Four.

There are, however, problems with the use of any medication or hormones. They include:

Possible Side Effects. Bleeding irregularities are fairly common with progesterone, and more serious side effects are possible. Chronic inflammation or ulceration of the digestive tract can be caused by the antiprostaglandins.

Necessity of Frequent Medical Visits for Some Women. Treatment can be very expensive. A doctor's prescription and careful follow-up are mandatory when using drugs.

Symptoms Are Controlled Only As Long As You're on the Medication. Since PMS is a long-term problem that becomes worse with age, for many women this can mean ten to twenty-five years of taking a drug or hormone. Many women either don't want to or can't be on medication for the remainder of their menstruating years.

For Many Women, Medication Does Not Offer a Complete Cure. I have seen many patients who have excellent relief of cramps with the use of the antiprostaglandins but are still left with their other symptoms.

Many of my patients do choose to use progesterone or the antiprostaglandins. Most of them, however, work toward getting off medication within a three-to-nine-month period. I hope that if you have to have drug treatment, you will work to get off it, too.

Conclusion

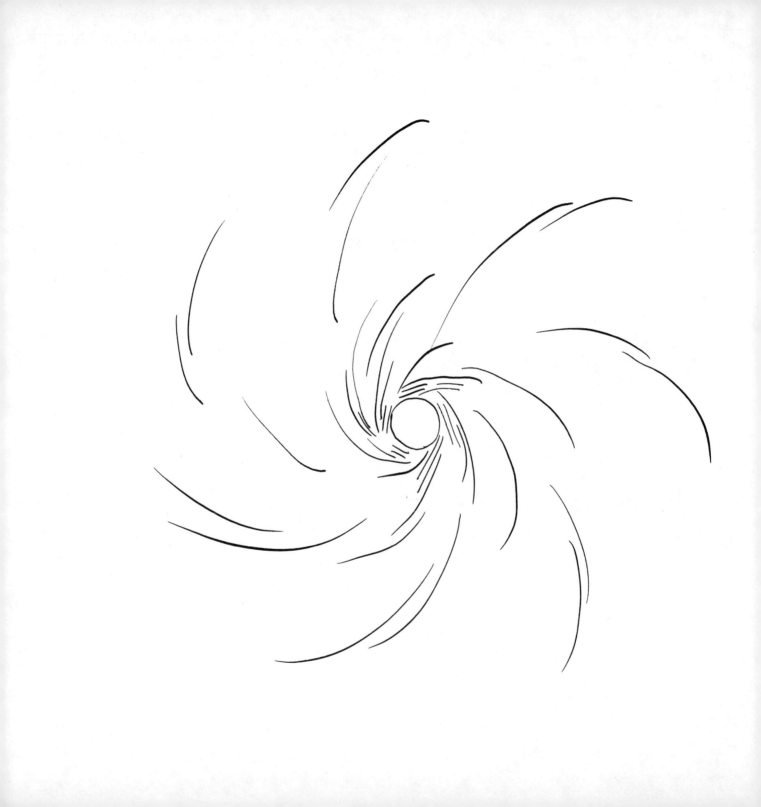

18

Making Your Program Work

The Complete Treatment Chart on page 60 should help you put together your own program simply and easily. It emphasizes all the main points that I would like you to keep in mind. Don't get bogged down in details. Always keep in mind your ultimate objective: *relief of PMS.*

Enjoy the program. Have fun with the exercises. Treat the changes in your dietary habits as an opportunity to try delicious new foods.

Healing occurs in a stepwise progression. It is never a straight line. Don't feel guilty if you miss a day of exercises. Don't become discouraged if you go off your diet for holidays, vacations, or just because your old food cravings become too strong. Everyone falls down at times. The successful person picks herself up and moves on. Just keep going back to your goals periodically and review the general guidelines that I've outlined for you.

Be your own best feedback system. Become sensitive to your body's messages. Your body will tell you when certain foods or emotional stress triggers PMS.

Remember that even moderate changes in your habits can relieve PMS.

Nutrition

Make all nutritional changes gradually. Review the lists of foods to limit and foods to emphasize periodically. Each time you review this list, pick several more foods that you are willing to eliminate or try. Review these lists as often as you choose, but try to do it on a regular basis. Every small change that you make in your diet can help.

Review the guidelines for each meal. You may want to restructure a particular meal. The sample menus that I've provided in the text can serve as models for you.

Use vitamin and herbal supplements during the premenstrual period to help round out your nutritional needs. Both are very helpful for control of your PMS.

Stress Reduction

Your stress reduction exercises will help to change your belief system about your body as well as improve your autonomic nervous system function.

When you begin your program, set aside half an hour for several consecutive days and try all the stress reduction exercises described in this book. Find the combination that works for you and then practice it regularly.

The exercises should be done on a daily basis for at least a few minutes a day. You may find that the best times to practice them are in the morning when you wake up or at night before you go to sleep. Other useful times are during the day when you are feeling particularly frazzled or stressed. Simply take ten minutes, close the door to your room, and relax. Deep-breathe, meditate or use the PMS visualization or affirmations. You will find that you feel much better afterward. You may also find that you enjoy doing the stress-reduction exercises before doing your regular physical exercise.

Exercise

Moderate exercise—walking, jogging, swimming, playing tennis, or bicycling—should be done on a regular basis. Every day or every other day is best.

Specific PMS Corrective Exercises:
Acupressure Massage, Yoga, Neurolymphatic Points, Neurovascular Holding Points

The first week or two, set aside half an hour to an hour a day for several consecutive days and do the exercises that warm up, tone, and energize the entire body. Find the ones you enjoy the most. These should always precede any specific corrective exercises for your symptoms. Find the combination of warm-ups and exercises that works best for you.

Look up the specific exercises that will correct your symptoms on the Complete Treatment Chart (page 60). Try out all of the exercises for your specific symptoms. Find the ones that work best for you.

Practice them on a regular basis. Starting them a few days before your PMS begins will help to prevent the symptoms.

Workbook Section

Use your workbook section on a regular basis. It will make the program much easier and more effective for you.

The workbook pages give you a structured format with which to evaluate your habit patterns, your symptoms, and your success. The habit evaluation section will show you which areas of your life contribute to your symptoms. Check off your symptoms during the premenstrual period and list which treatments you are doing during this period to help correct them. It is important that you give yourself this feedback in an organized and easy-to-use format.

Conclusion

I've told you all I know about a self-help approach to PMS. I hope this information will be of help to you. I've enjoyed writing this book and I hope that you can achieve the same wonderful results that I and my patients have had. Practice good nutritional habits, relaxation and stress reduction techniques, moderate exercise, and any specific corrective techniques that work for you to relieve your specific symptoms. Most of all, enjoy your life each and every day.

Sources for Further Help and Information

Support Groups

PMS Action is a women's group that helps disseminate information about PMS. You can get in touch with them at:

PMS Action
P.O. Box 9326
Madison, WI 53715
(608) 274-6688

To find out about local support groups in your community, contact:

The National PMS Society
P.O. Box 11467
Durham, NC 27703

Cookbooks

There are a few good cookbooks with recipes that can be adapted by women with PMS. They do have some forbidden ingredients, but when you come to one, you can look back at the list of substitutions I've suggested and use one of them instead. Or you may simply want to use ingredients in the recipe and call the dish that you are preparing a treat.

Michel Abehsera, *Cooking with Care and Purpose* (Brooklyn, NY: Swan House Publishing, 1978).

———, *Zen Macrobiotic Cooking* (New York: Avon, 1968).

Wendy Esko, *Introducing Macrobiotic Cooking* (Tokyo: Japan Publications Inc., 1978).

JoAnne Levitt, Linda Smith, and Christine Warren, *Kripalu Kitchen* (Summit Station, PA: Kripalu Publications, 1980).

Ruth Ann Manners and William Manners, *The Quick and Easy Vegetarian Cookbook* (New York: M. Evans, 1978).

Nathan Pritikin, *The Pritikin Permanent Weight Loss Manual* (New York: Bantam, 1982).

Laurel Robertson, Carol Flinders, and Bronwen Godfrey, *Laurel's Kitchen* (New York: Bantam, 1978).

Craig and Ann Sams, *The Brown Rice Cookbook* (Wellingborough, Northhamptonshire, England: Thorsons Publishers, Ltd., 1980.)

Sources for Hard-to-Find Foods and Products

If stores near you don't carry the foods mentioned in this chapter, you may be able to order them by mail from one of the following:

Dr. Hazel Parcell
1605 Coal Avenue S.E.
Albuquerque, NM 87106
(mail order source for Biosalt)

Erehwon Natural Foods
236 Washington Street
Brookline, MA 02146
(free catalogue of many foods, herbs and spices)

Grain Country
3448 30th Street
San Diego, CA 92104
(714) 298-1052
(complete line of macrobiotic food, produce, utensils, and books)

Mountain Ark Trading Company
Macrobiotic Mail Order
109 South East Street
Fayetteville, AR 72701
(501) 442-7191
(nationwide mail and phone orders)

Help in Managing Stress

Books

Norman Shealy, M.D., *Ninety Days to Self Health* (New York: Bantam Books, 1977).

Shakti Gawain, *Creative Visualization* (New York: Bantam Books, 1978).

Hans Selye, *Stress Without Distress* (New York: Signet, 1975).

Tapes

"Stress Reduction Tape for PMS," PMS Self-Help Center, 170 State St., Suite 222, Los Altos, CA 94022

Alphanetic Series, ten-tape set, Life Dynamics Fellowship, 2704 So. Grand, Santa Ana, CA 92705

"Creative Visualization," Shakti Gawain, Whatever
Publishing Co., 158 E. Blithedale Ave., Mill Valley,
CA 94941

"Stress Reduction and Creative Meditation," Marcus
Allen, Whatever Publishing Co., 158 E. Blithedale
Ave., Mill Valley, CA 94941

"Two Inner Journeys to Tranquility," Earth Light
Sound, 13906 Ventura Blvd., Sherman Oaks, CA
91423

The PMS Self-Help Center

The PMS Self-Help Center was established to disseminate information about PMS and health aids for use at home
to help alleviate PMS symptoms. The health aids include: a
vitamin supplement; an herbal formulation; audio tapes for
relaxation; a videotape, or full-color slides, of the exercise
programs in this book; and a videotape of demonstrations of
the cooking techniques, foods, and food products described in this book.

The center offers seminars and workshops for health
professionals, corporations, and women who suffer from
PMS. It also offers continuing education classes for nurses.
Its large staff of physicians donate time for lectures on PMS
self-help to women's groups and clinics.

For women who need further guidance, the center can arrange for full clinical services.

The PMS Self-Help Center
170 State St., Suite 222
Los Altos, CA 94022
(800) 227-3900; (800) 632-2122 from California
Susan M. Lark, M.D., director
Christine Green, M.D., director of patient education.

Suggested Readings for Women with PMS

Acupuncture

The Academy of Traditional Chinese Medicine. *An Outline of Chinese Acupuncture*. New York: Pergamon Press, 1975.

Bendix, G. *Stress Point Therapy*. New York: Avon, 1976.

Carter, Mildred. *Hand Reflexology*. West Nyack, NY: Parker Publishing Co., 1975.

Chan, P. C. *Acupressure Self-Help Therapy for Menstrual Pain*. Monterey, CA: Chinese Total Health Center, 1980.

———. *Ear Acupressure*. Monterey, CA: Chan's Corporation, 1977.

———. *Essentials of Acupressure Therapy*. Monterey, CA: Chinese Total Health Center, 1980.

———. *Finger Acupressure*. Los Angeles: Price/Stern/Sloan, 1982.

Gach, Michael Reed, and Carolyn Marco. *Acu-Yoga*. Tokyo: Japan Publications, 1981.

Ingham, Eunice. *Stories the Feet Have Told*. St. Petersburg, FL: Ingham Publishers, 1963.

Kaye, Ann, and Don C. Matchan. *Reflexology for Good Health*. North Hollywood, CA: Wilshire Book Company, 1978.

Teeguarden, Iona. *Acupressure Way of Health: Jin Shin Do*. Tokyo: Japan Publications, 1978.

Wensel, Louis. *Acupuncture for Americans*. Reston, VA: Reston Publishing Company, 1980.

Exercise

Harrison, Michelle, M.D. *Self-Help for Premenstrual Syndrome*. Cambridge, MA: Matrix Press, 1982.

Kraus, Hans, M.D. *Backache, Stress and Tension*. New York: Simon & Schuster, 1965.

Letvin, Maggie. *Maggie's Woman's Book*. Boston: Houghton Mifflin, 1980.

Michele, Arthur, M.D. *Orthotherapy*. New York: M. Evans, 1972.

Storch, Marcia, M.D., with Carrie Carmichael. *How to Relieve Cramps and Other Menstrual Problems*. New York: Workman Publishing Company, 1982.

Nutrition and Cooking

Abehsera, Michel. *Cooking with Care and Purpose*. Brooklyn, NY: Swan House Publishing, 1978.

———. *Zen Macrobiotic Cooking*. New York: Avon, 1968.

Abraham, Guy E. "The Calcium Controversy." *Journal of Applied Nutrition* 34(2):69–73 (Fall, 1982).

Abraham, G. E., U. D. Schwartz, and M. M. Lubran. "Effect of Vitamin B_6 on Plasma and Red Cell Magnesium Levels in Premenopausal Women." *Annals of Clinical Laboratory Science* 2(4): 333–336 (July-August, 1981).

Abraham, Guy E., and Joel T. Hargrove. "Effect of Vitamin B_6 on Premenstrual Symptomology in Women with Premenstrual Tension Syndromes: A Double-Blind Crossover Study." *Infertility* 3:155 (1980).

Abraham, Guy E., Charlotte Elsner, and Linda Lucas. "Hormonal and Behaviorial Changes during the Menstrual Cycle." *Senologia* 3:33-38 (1978).

Abraham, Guy E., and M. M. Lubran. "Serum and Red Cell Magnesium Levels in Patients with Premenstrual Tension." *American Journal of Clinical Nutrition* 34:2364–2366 (1981).

Christopher, John R. *School of Natural Healing*. Provo, UT: BiWorld Publishers, 1976.

Goei, G. S., and G. E. Abraham. "Effect of a Nutritional Supplement, Optivite, on Premenstrual Symptomology in Patients with Premenstrual Tension." *Journal of Reproductive Medicine* (in press).

Hargrove, J. T., and G. E. Abraham. "Effect of Vitamin B_6 on Infertility in Women with Premenstrual Tension." *Infertility* 2:315–322 (1979).

Hargrove, J. T., and G. E. Abraham. "The Incidence of Premenstrual Tension in a Gynecological Clinic." *Journal of Reproductive Medicine* (in press).

Holick, M. F., and M. B. Clark. "The Photogenesis and Metabolism of Vitamin D." *Federation Proceedings* 37:2567–2574 (1978).

Kushi, Aveline Tomoko. *How to Cook with Miso*. Tokyo: Japan Publications, 1978.

Levitt, JoAnn, Linda Smith, and Christine Warren. *Kripalu Kitchen*. Summit Station, PA: Kripalu Publications, 1980.

Lucas, Richard. *Secrets of the Chinese Herbalists*. West Nyack, NY: Parker Publishing, 1977.

Manners, Ruth Ann, and William Manners. *The Quick and Easy Vegetarian Cookbook.* New York: M. Evans, 1978.

Pritikin, Nathan. *The Pritikin Permanent Weight-Loss Manual.* New York: Bantam, 1982.

Raymond, Jennifer. *The Best of Jenny's Kitchen.* New York: Avon, 1980.

Royal, Penny C. *Herbally Yours.* Provo, UT: BiWorld Publishers, 1976.

Sams, Craig, and Ann Sams. *The Brown Rice Cookbook.* Wellingborough, Northamptonshire, England: Thorsons Publishers, Ltd., 1980.

Seelig, M. S. "The Requirement of Magnesium by the Normal Adult." *American Journal of Clinical Nutrition* 14: 342 (1964).

Weber, Marcea. *The Sweet Life Natural Macrobiotic Desserts.* Tokyo: Japan Publications, 1981.

Wright, Jonathan V. *Dr. Wright's Book of Nutritional Therapy.* Emmaus, PA: Rodale Press, 1979.

Women's Books

Budoff, Penny W., M.D. *No More Menstrual Cramps and Other Good News.* New York: Penguin, 1980.

Cooke, Cynthia W., M.D., and Susan Dworkin. *The Ms. Guide to a Woman's Health.* New York: Anchor Books, 1979.

Kistner, Robert W., M.D. *Gynecology: Principles and Practice.* Chicago: Year Book Medical Publishers, 1971.

Lauersen, Niels, M.D., and Steven Whitney. *It's Your Body: A Woman's Guide to Gynecology.* New York: Playboy Press, 1977.

Seaman, Barbara, and Gideon Seaman, M.D. *Women and the Crisis in Sex Hormones.* New York: Rawson Associates, 1977.

Yoga

Moore, Marcia, and Mark Douglas. *Yoga.* Arcane, ME: Arcane Publications, 1967.

Stearn, Jess. *Yoga, Youth, and Reincarnation.* New York: Bantam Books, 1965.

Reviews

Abraham, Guy E. "The Normal Menstrual Cycle" in *Endocrine Causes of Menstrual Disorders*, ed. J. R. Givens, M.D. Chicago: Year Book Medical Publishers, 1977.

————. "Premenstrual Tension" in *Current Problems in Obstetrics and Gynecology.* Chicago: Yearbook Medical Publishers, 1980.

————. "Primary Dysmenorrhea." *Clinical Obstetrics and Gynecology* 21:139 (1978).

Reid, R. L., and S. S. C. Yen. "Premenstrual Syndrome." *American Journal of Obstetrics and Gynecology* 139:85–104 (1981).

Tonks, C. M. *Premenstrual Tension. British Journal of Psychiatry* Special Publication No. 9 (1975).

Index

About the Author

Susan M. Lark, M.D., is a diplomate of the American Academy of Family Physicians, with a medical degree from Northwestern University. She was the founder and medical director of the South Drive Medical Clinic in Mountain View, California, and of the Northern California Premenstrual Clinic, where she treated hundreds of women with PMS. She also has been clinical instructor at Stanford Medical School's Department of Family and Preventive Medicine. She is currently associate member of the Department of Family Medicine, El Camino Hospital in Mountain View, California, and director of the PMS Self-Help Center in Los Altos, California.